WHAT'S NEW ABOUT THIS EDITION?

Overall

The first version of this book invited anyone to participate in the rich culture of the marathon, with a highly successful training program that allows for carrying on family, career, and social life.

This new revised version takes it further, providing tools to manage fatigue, eliminate injury, ensure proper pacing, and adjust for heat—setting realistic goals and monitoring progress, while receiving all of the satisfaction and achievement of running a marathon.

Pacing

- My new "magic mile" time trial predicts a top performance extremely accurately during a season.
- Based upon tens of thousands: new data comparing the per mile slowdown that occurs from one mile to 26 miles
- Each runner is told how to pick a safe pace for the long run.
- A new rule of thumb for slowdown due to heat: 30 seconds a mile slower for every 5°F increase above 60°F (20 sec/ kilometer for every 2°C above 14°C)

Walk Breaks

- Since first publishing this book, the percentage of marathoners using walk breaks has increased from 20% to 40%, and is growing every year.
- During the last decade, I've found much more successful run-walk-run ratios that produce faster times.
- In this version of the book I explain how to set up the right ratio for the individual, through use of the "magic mile."
- Run-walk-run ratios are broken down by pace per mile.
- New stories about success with walk breaks

Nutrition

- How to use certain websites (some free) to gain control over nutrition
- Use of these sites allows each person to know if he/she is getting the nutrients needed.
- Fat burning can be done while training for a marathon if the run-walk-run ratio is liberal enough on the walking side.
- A rule of thumb on how many calories to ingest to maintain blood sugar level
- Guidance on fluid intake to keep water flowing through the system
- How to avoid *hyponatremia* (a condition that kills marathoners each year and is preventable) by controlling the quantity of fluid during long runs and marathons

Motivation

- How to train yourself to be motivated
- Techniques for exercising when you're not motivated
- How to keep going when you don't feel up to it
- Quick fixes that can keep runners motivated during the latter stages of the marathon

The Training Schedule

- Adjustments have been made to the weekly schedule to reduce injuries and improve performance.
- Time goal runners will add to the number of mile repetitions.
- Walk break guidelines for the mile repetition speedwork
- Acceleration gliders and cadence drills are now in the schedule.
- "Race Rehearsal" segments are inserted into some of the weekday runs for time goal runners.

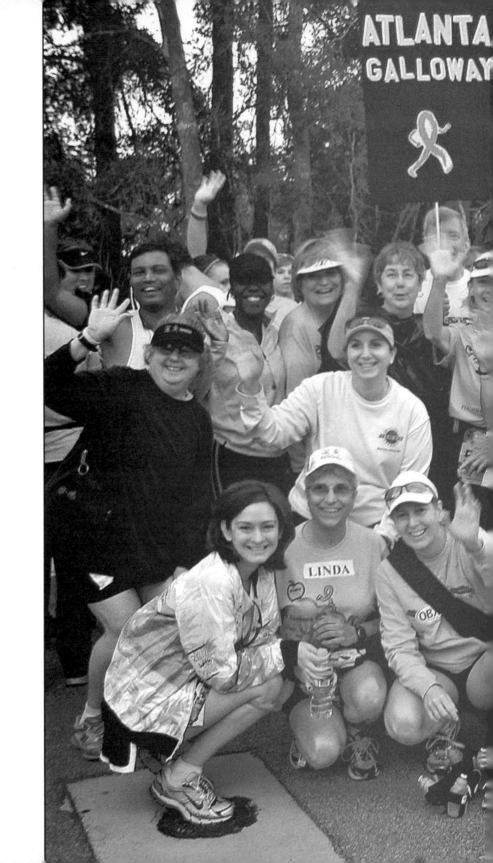

MARATHON

YOU CAN DO IT!

JEFF GALLOWAY

Distributed in the United States by Publishers Group West and in Canada by Publishers Group Canada.

Library of Congress Cataloging-in-Publication Data

Galloway, Jeff, 1945–
   Marathon : you can do it! / Jeff Galloway. — Rev. ed.
      p.   cm.
   Includes index.
   ISBN 978-0-936070-48-3
   1. Marathon running—Training.   I. Title.
   GV1065.17.T73G35 2010
   796.42′52—dc22

                                               2010009858

6 5 4 3 2 1—14 13 12 11 10
(Lowest digits indicate number and year of latest printing.)

Printed in the United States of America

Shelter Publications, Inc.
P. O. Box 279
Bolinas, California 94924
415-868-0280
E-mail: shelter@shelterpub.com
Orders, toll-free: 1-800-307-0131

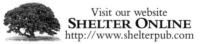

Visit our website
SHELTER ONLINE
http://www.shelterpub.com

Photos front and back cover by Joseph Sohm, *Visions of America*

PREFACE

"Jeff Galloway is one of those rare individuals who not only knows his craft, but also has the ability to convey this knowledge through teaching."

–Frank Shorter

There's a second running revolution going on in America these days.

The first was in the early '70s, launched by Frank Shorter's gold medal in the '72 Olympic marathon, and by a group of exciting new American runners: Bill Rodgers, Steve Prefontaine, Don Kardong, Amby Burfoot, Jeff Galloway, and others. An astonishing number of (mostly baby-boom) people took to the streets and roads in those years, races proliferated, and what had been an off-beat sport for a relatively few hardcore endurance athletes became a national craze for millions of Americans.

The second revolution has quietly taken place, with less fanfare, over the last ten or so years: People are running marathons in unprecedented numbers. Marathon participation has quadrupled since the late '70s.

What's going on here? Why has this happened?

There's a new attitude among the new marathoners. Whereas in the '70s and '80s, the new runners trained hard and seriously—"pedal to the metal"—and went after "PRs" (personal records), today's marathoners are in it for the fun. Their focus is on finishing a marathon. They're not trying to win their age group; their goal is to finish. They're not into drastic weight loss; they're in it for the fun, the companionship, and the achievement. It's a different attitude, and it's allowed literally hundreds of thousands of people to have life-enriching experiences.

No one has promoted this change of attitude among runners more than Olympian Jeff Galloway. Jeff started his Galloway training programs in the mid-1970s, and published his best-selling *Galloway's Book on Running* in 1984 (in nine languages, over 700,000 copies sold). Then in 2001 he wrote the first edition of *Marathon: You Can Do It!* in which he promoted a more relaxed, gentler training program, the secret ingredient being his run-walk-run method.

In the Galloway program, you take walk breaks during your training runs *and* during the marathon itself. Since the first edition 10 years ago, the percentage of marathoners taking walk breaks has increased from 20% to over 40%.

Jeff has coached over 100,000 runners since the first edition, and he has modified this revised edition to incorporate what he's learned. *(See page 1 for a summary of what's new in this book.)*

Jeff now has marathon training programs in 81 cities. He has a blog, a Twitter account (with over 7000 followers), and two Facebook accounts. *(See p. 199 for the web addresses.)*

In the following pages, Jeff lays out his training programs *(flip ahead to pages 35 to 57 for a preview)*, and offers his tips and insights on all aspects of preparing for a marathon. Whatever your athletic ability, with help from Jeff, you can likely achieve your dream of completing a marathon. Read on!

–Lloyd Kahn, Editor

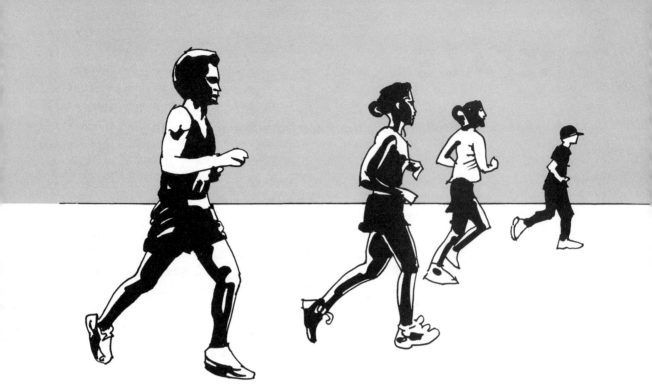

CONTENTS

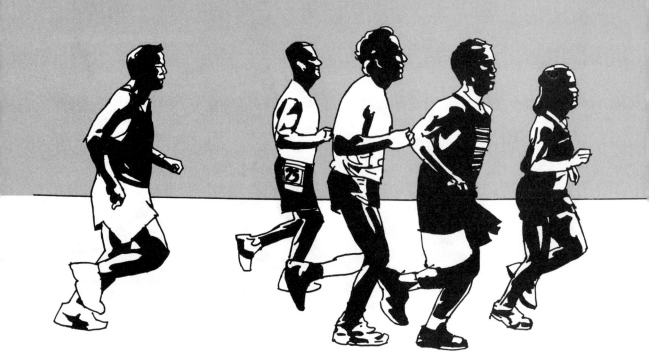

INTRODUCTION

WHY CHOOSE THE MARATHON?

There's been an overwhelming flood tide of entrants into marathons in the past few years. Beginning exercisers by the thousands are targeting a marathon instead of the safer choice of a 5K or 10K. Established marathons are filling their quotas earlier than ever, and in 2008, over 425,000 people finished a marathon—an all-time record. What started as a once-in-a-lifetime achievement is now being attained by former couch potatoes every six to twelve months.

At the same time that a majority of the North American population has been labeled "significantly overweight," marathon training has been designated as the fastest growing type of exercise. More than two million people train for a marathon each year; surely some start with the goal of losing weight. The overwhelming number of those who continue, however, do so because of the unequaled positive boost in attitude, significant stress release, and overall increase in vitality, focus and creativity.

As the average age of the marathoner has increased to 40+, the marathon has become a mid-life mission, an attainable goal. It could be worse: when you list the other mid-life diversions, the marathon's not a bad choice. At this stage of life, a high percentage of these first-time marathoners are accustomed to relying upon key people and leveraging influence through contacts, income and other negotiable items. The marathon stands out as one of the most esteemed of life's achievements, but it has to be won by pulling from within oneself physical, mental, and spiritual resources over an extended period of time. Universal respect flows from sedentary observers who wish they could find the fortitude to get out there and do the same. Participants discover a mature self-respect, along with previously dormant strength to meet the challenges of this six-month adventure.

Part of the fulfillment must come from getting back to our roots. Our ancient ancestors walked and ran for thousands of miles each year to survive. In the process, they developed and passed on to us a treasury of physical and mental skills, which we renew on every run. The challenge of a significant physical journey on foot unleashes some primitive connections to our identity as human beings.

Most new marathoners bypass shorter distance events because they know that they need a challenging mission. By writing the marathon date on a calendar, one becomes more motivated to get out the door when the alarm goes off way too early or on days when the weather is bad.

If you have read this far, chances are you're ready to go forward with one of the most fulfilling experiences of your life. At the very least, you're saying that you want to take responsibility for your health and your attitude. On the long list of benefits from such a program, those two are at the top.

Every marathoner, no matter how experienced, has to dig down and find resources to get through the training program and to finish the marathon. You'll discover strengths that you didn't know were there. Most of those on a marathon mission become more positive and react more directly to life's offerings. When the finish banner comes into view and you realize the end of your journey is near, even the tough guys let loose some tears.

Over the past four decades, I've run over 150 marathons. I've received the same wonderful exhilaration when running them fast (2:16) as I do when running them slowly.

To reach the finish line in a marathon is to enter an elite group: only about one-tenth of 1 percent of the population does it.

By the way, my most treasured marathon was my slowest. I ran with my father (age 75) in the 1996 Boston Marathon in 5:59:48. He tells folks that if I hadn't been there to slow him down, he'd have run much faster.

- To stick with a marathon training program for six months is to become a winner.
- To finish a marathon will leave you feeling like a champion!
- You can do it!

BEFORE YOU TAKE THOSE FIRST STEPS...

There are a very few people who should not exercise because of cardiovascular, structural, muscular, or other problems. It's very important to ensure that you are not in this risk category.

- Before beginning any exercise, diet or other improvement program, be sure to have yourself and the program evaluated by specialists in the areas you are pursuing.
- Your own specific body type and any physical problems may require program modifications.
- Always back off when you feel that the training may lead to an injury or health problems.
- Benefits come from regular exercise and steady adherence to a long-term program.
- Never radically increase the amount of exercise or drastically change your diet.
- The advice in this book is offered as such—advice from one exerciser to another. It is not meant to be a prescription.
- Joining a group helps motivation.
- Have FUN and you'll want to continue.

ORIGIN OF THE MARATHON

Over 2500 years ago, a lone runner sped through the Greek countryside to announce an unexpected Athenian victory over Persian forces in the Battle of Marathon.

But like so many supposedly simple historical facts, this one has many plots and subplots.

Marathon is a sunny, wind-swept coastal plain in northern Greece. There, in 490 B.C., the Athenian Army routed the numerically superior invading Persian Army in one of the most important battles in Western Civilization.

In 507 B.C., the Athenians asked King Darius I of Persia to form an alliance against their rival city-state to the north, the militaristic Sparta. In exchange, Athens was to be ruled by Darius. The Athenian government later rescinded the agreement, but Darius still considered himself the rightful ruler of Athens.

Around 500 B.C., Greeks living under Persian rule in Asia Minor (now Turkey) revolted against the Persians. The Athenians sent soldiers and ships to help the rebels, then attacked and burned Sardis, Darius'

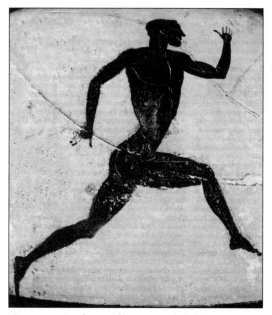

A runner in the stadion *race (a 200-meter sprint) in the ancient Greek Olympics. Note the long stride and high-swinging arms.*

capital in Asia Minor. Darius vowed revenge, pledging to conquer Athens.

In 490 B.C., the Persians set out with an army of 20,000 troops and 200 ships for Athens. They invaded Greek soil and set up camp at Marathon, about 25 miles northeast of Athens.

This was a crucial period in the development of the democratic experiment in Athens. Unlike the more autocratic governments of the other great civilizations to that point, the Athenians encouraged individual freedom and personal growth and achievement. The epitome of this philosophy was the Olympic games, which elevated fitness and sport to a level of respect equal to that of valued professions. Indeed, the Greeks recorded history according to the four-year Olympiad in which the event occurred.

The historical record of this period was passed down in oral reports and written more than two centuries later by Herodotus and others. While the storytelling tradition in Greek history has been shown to be generally accurate through later research and excavation, names and details sometimes become blurred. There are differing accounts of all this, but some threads of truth seem to appear in most versions of the battle. What follows is my assessment of what happened after studying many different historical accounts of the Battle of Marathon.

When the committee of three generals in charge of Athenian forces received reports of the massive beachhead of Persians at Marathon, they decided to send a messenger

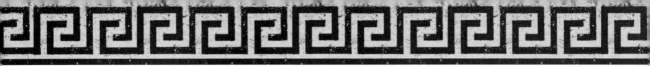

to Sparta for help. Although Athens and Sparta were not on best of terms, Sparta would benefit from an Athenian victory; without it, the Persians would be heading their way.

The Athenian generals knew this was a winner-take-all situation. If they lost, the Persians would kill them, loot and burn Athens, and enslave their families. The residents of Athens already had a plan to burn the city if necessary in order to deprive the Persians of some of the spoils.

The generals chose a runner from the cult of Greek messengers known as *hemerodromoi* (all-day runners) to deliver a message to Sparta. These were professional long-distance runners who never competed. Rather they provided fast communication links throughout the country. Often logging more than a marathon distance a day, these endurance specialists could navigate the tricky Greek terrain, covering very long distances faster than horses. They were expected not only to deliver the news but also to interpret it, emphasize key points, and return with a reply, including a description of the facial expression and emotion of the respondent.

The messenger sent to Sparta was probably *Phidippides* (there are different versions of his name), and the distance was 147 miles. Phidippides reached Sparta in about a day-and-a-half, a magnificent feat over hilly terrain.* He went before the Spartan rulers to plead for their help. Relatively quickly, they gave him the good news that Sparta would send troops. Unfortunately, however, they were in the middle of a community ritual and couldn't come for about ten days.

Another day and a half later, Phidippides had run back to the hills above Marathon and reported to his leaders. Some 250 miles on foot in less than a week!

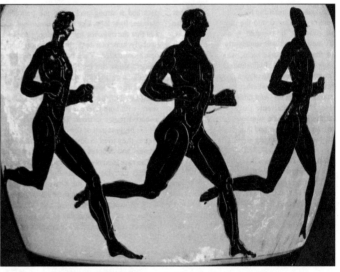

Depiction of runners in the dolichos, *a long-distance (2000 meters) race. Note the short stride and minimal arm-swing as compared to the sprinter on the previous page.* (The British Museum, London)

---

*Phidippides' historic run is commemorated each year with the 147.2-mile Spartathalon ultra-distance run, from Athens to Sparta. The course today follows pavement and gravel roads during the hot time of year, and goes over a mountain range near the 100-mile point. The event is usually won in around 26 hours these days, but the course record is an incredible 21:51, set in 1983 by the Greek ultra-distance champion, Yiannis Kouros.

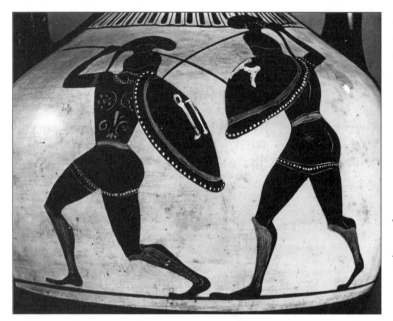

Scene of the hoplomachia *event in the Olympics, a duel between two contestants wearing heavy armor.* (Museo Arquelogico Nacional, Madrid)

The illustrations in this history section are from amphora, *two-handled vases awarded to winners in the ancient Olympic games. They were filled with olive oil and were painted with the athletic event in which the winning athlete participated.*

Realizing that the Persians wouldn't wait ten days to attack, the Athenians advanced to Marathon, where they encamped and waited. The Persians waited too. Part of the Persian strategy was for their allies in Athens to start a civil war to weaken the city, and in a few days they loaded part of their forces onto ships and set sail for Athens.

Seeing their chance for victory, the Athenians devised an innovative battle plan and attacked the Persian troops left at Marathon with a thin front line. The Persians quickly broke through to the center

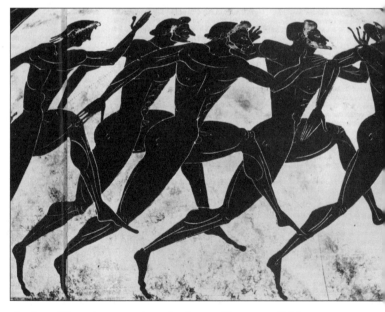

Ancient Olympic competitors in the stadion *race (200-meter sprint). Note the wide stride and vigorous arm-swings.* (Metropolitan Museum, New York)

of the battlefield, thought they had won, and started celebrating. Suddenly the Greeks attacked with their best soldiers in inward-wheeling wings and surrounded the Persians. Having lost their focus and probably suspecting a supernatural force, the Persians fled. By the time they made it back to their ships, they had lost 6,400 men; the Greeks lost 192. The battle is said to have proved the superiority of the Greek long spears, swords, and armor over the Persians' weapons. (And also superior strategy!)

History tells us that Phidippides was then sent from Marathon to Athens to announce the victory. He had to cover the distance as quickly as possible since the Athenians were prepared to burn the city if defeat looked imminent. Phidippides sped the 25-mile distance to Athens and collapsed with his unexpected but now-famous word of victory, *Nenikhkamen* (pronounced *Nenikékamen*) or *Nike*, meaning: "We have won." Athens would live but the exhausted (and perhaps wounded) messenger would die.

In the first modern Olympic games in Athens in 1896, it was suggested that Phidippides' victory run be commemorated in a footrace from the Plain of Marathon to the Olympic stadium in Athens. The distance from the tomb at the battlefield to the stadium was 25 miles, and this continued as the official distance until the London Olympics in 1908. The 25-mile course had been measured out and marked when the Queen (Alexandra, wife of Edward VII) asked if she might be able to watch the start from Windsor Castle. The course was extended by 1.2 miles to accommodate the royal request, and the new distance

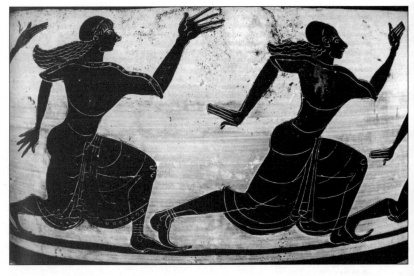

The Heraia *were Greek games for women, held in conjunction with the men's Olympics. Women ran a 160-meter race in tunics, with loose hair, and were divided into three groups according to age. Hera was a Greek goddess who was worshiped in a temple in Olympia two centuries before the construction of the temple of Zeus.* (Musei Vaticani, Rome)

became official. Today's marathon is 26 miles, 385 yards. The marathon is one of two events that has been run in every one of the modern Olympic games.

It's interesting to note that in the first Olympic marathon in 1896, the competitors ran *and walked* in the race.

Ancient Greek Olympians ran short-distance races in stadiums. Each year I have the good fortune to take groups of runners and walkers to visit these sites in Greece, when we run the Athens Marathon. I still get chills every time I visit and jog down the field. You can put your feet in the grooves of the starting blocks used by ancient runners and experience a direct connection to the vitality of the ancient Olympic concept.

This will keep you motivated to get out the door for weeks or months on your return home!

A few years ago, as I was walking from the 1896 stadium towards the ancient site of Athens, I realized that Phidippides would have run about 26 miles—the ancient town of Athens is about a mile further down the road from where the first Olympic marathon ended in 1896.

A tradition among veteran marathoners when passing the original finish distance at 25 miles is to say "God save the Queen" or something like that. But considering Phidippides' run for reinforcements to Sparta and back, today's marathoners are getting off easy—we could be running 260 miles!

TRAINING

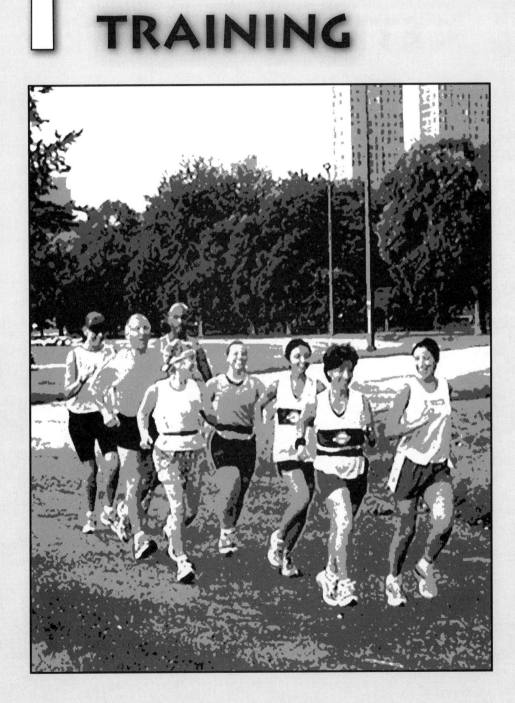

1 GETTING STARTED

THE BASICS OF YOUR MARATHON PROGRAM

The marathon is primarily an endurance event. It is only secondarily a race and should not be an ordeal. This isn't to say it's a walk in the park, but you should be able to finish a marathon, enjoy the sense of achievement it gives you, and look forward to running your next one. The Galloway program will enable you to do just that, all in about six months. The purpose of the program is to build endurance at a steady incremental rate without subjecting your body to stress and injury. Key components are persistence and moderation. The unique factor introduced in this program is *the run-walk-run method*. As you will see, short walks interspersed with your training runs will prevent you from pushing yourself to exhaustion and injury.

At the beginning, the program is very simple (you *run* just three days a week), as shown below:

In summary, you:

- Walk for 30–60 minutes three days a week
- Run for 30 minutes (with walk breaks) twice a week
- Take one day off to rest
- Take a long run (with walk breaks) once a week (or once every other week)

Bare-bones program

Even if you only have 60 minutes to exercise during the work week, you can start training for the marathon. The minimum is actually better for insuring against injuries. *To start with the bare minimum, you run/walk 30 minutes twice a week.* Then you can work into long runs, starting at 3 miles and gradually increasing by an average of one mile each week until it reaches 10 miles. Then, you'll do the long run every other week, with a run/walk of half the distance on alternate "off" weekends. Once you've completed the 17-miler, you'll receive two weekends off for good behavior, shifting to a long run every third week. *(See pp. 36–37.)*

THE THREE-DAY-A-WEEK PROGRAM
Goal: To Finish

Mon*	Tue	Wed*	Thu	Fri*	Sat	Sun*
Walk 30–60 min	Run/walk 30 min	Walk 30–60 min	Run/walk 30 min	Walk 30–60 min	Off	Long run/walk

*optional at beginning

Some running terminology

First let's define some running terms:

Cross training: Exercise other than running. Cycling, swimming, or weight training are typical cross training activities for runners; these sports develop different muscles. Cross training may not improve your marathon time, nor is it necessary for you to finish a marathon, but it will provide attitude-boosting endorphins, stress release, and burn fat on non-running days.

Form work: When you concentrate on form while training. There are a lot of components here, but three of the most important to focus on are: **c**hest up (good posture), **h**ips forward, and **p**ushing off strongly with your feet. (Think **C-H-P.**)

Hill training: Running hills prepares your muscles for running faster; there is less pounding and therefore less muscle strain than running on the flat.

Long run: The most important component of your marathon training. The beginner starts with a 3-mile run, gradually building to a 26-mile run three weeks before the marathon. You use walk breaks on all the long runs.

Maintenance runs: The short runs, taken twice a week and lasting no longer than an hour, that consolidate the endurance gains acquired during the previous week's long run.

Rest: Rest is as important a factor in your training as is running. Without adequate rest you will injure your muscles, possibly beyond repair in time for the race. During the week, you rest while training by taking walk breaks and you also rest by not training for longer than 60 minutes at a time.

Resting allows your muscles to rebuild stronger than they were before.

Run: A run is a run. It is not a sprint; it is a steady run, but not a continuous run, since you will be using walk breaks to rest and rejuvenate your muscles.

Speed work: Here you run measured one-milers at a specified time *(as designated in the programs on pp. 36–57).* Speed training is time-consuming, and recommended for competitive runners, not first-time marathoners.

Two-Minute Rule: You run all your long runs at least 2 minutes slower per mile than you could run a marathon as predicted by the "magic mile" time trial. You will get the same endurance benefits running slowly as you would running faster. However you'll recover much faster from running slowly.

Walk: A walk is a walk. In this program you walk before you run and you walk during runs. Start by walking 30 minutes a day. If you can't walk comfortably that long, take short breaks. Look at the scenery for a while, then continue. Gradually increase the distance of your walks until you're walking a maximum of 50 minutes, three days a week. Then stay at that level.

Walk break: Periods of walking taken on long runs. *This is your secret weapon.* Walk breaks allow your running muscles to recover before they are injured and conserve your energy so you can exercise for longer periods, which builds the endurance you need. In the beginning, your runs will actually be walks interspersed with short periods of running; over time, the running portions will become longer and the walk breaks shorter.

The "magic mile" time trial (MM)

1. Go to a track or other accurately measured course. One mile is 4 laps around a track.
2. Warm up by walking for 5 minutes, then running a minute and walking a minute for 6–10 minutes and then jogging an easy 800-meter (half mile or two laps around a track).
3. Do 4 acceleration gliders. *(See pp. 115–116.)*
4. Walk for 3–4 minutes.
5. Run fast—for you—for 4 laps. Use walk break suggestions in this chapter or run the way you want.
6. On your first time trial, don't run all-out from the start—just a little faster than you have been running.
7. Warm down by reversing the warmup.
8. A school track is the best venue. Don't use a treadmill because they tend to be notoriously uncalibrated and often tell you that you ran farther or faster than you really did.
9. On each successive test, try to adjust your pace in order to run a faster time than you've run before.
10. Use "Galloway's Performance Predictor" on p. 9 to see what time is predicted in the goal races.

Wall: "Hitting the wall" is a runner's phrase meaning that you get so tired you can barely go on, your reserves are depleted. These training programs will allow you to improve your endurance so you can cross the finish line without running up against "the wall."

The "Two-Minute Rule": On long runs, you must run at least 2 minutes per mile slower than you could run in a marathon as predicted by the "magic mile" time trial.

ENDURANCE (Long runs) + MAINTENANCE (Two 30-minute runs) + REST

Your body is designed to improve its endurance continuously if you gently stress it in a pattern of increases, rest enough for rebuilding, and do regular maintenance so that it won't forget the process. Think of your training program as a sound system. Each exercise session serves as a component designed to produce a specific effect. The long run gradually gets longer, and this develops the endurance necessary for finishing the marathon. The slow and minimal 60 minutes of maintenance run/walks during the week simply maintain the conditioning gained on the weekend. On other days it's crucial to allow the running muscles to rest—they need time to rebuild and they then make marvelous adaptations for easier and longer running.

The long run builds endurance

As you extend a mile or three farther on each long one, you push back your endurance limit. It's important to go slowly on each of these (at least two minutes per mile slower than your current marathon pace) to make it easy for your muscles to extend their current endurance limit and recover afterward. As you lengthen the long one to 26 miles, you build the exact endurance necessary to complete the marathon. Walk breaks, taken from the beginning (see section below) will also speed your recovery and make the extra distance on each run a gentle challenge.

Non-long-run weekends

On the alternate ("off") weekends, there are several options. Most runners will do a slow run of about half the distance of the current long run (up to 7 miles). On some of these "easy" weekends, run the "magic mile" to predict what you might be able to do in a marathon. *(See Predicting Race Performance on p. 187.)* Veterans will do speed sessions on some of the non-long-run weekends. If you're feeling good during these shorter runs, you can run them continuously, but there's no advantage in doing this. In other words, walk breaks are at your discretion on the shorter runs, including the ones during the week.

> Yes, it's possible to train for the marathon and have a life!

Walk breaks on long runs:

- Must be taken early and often to reduce pounding and fatigue
- Must be taken often to allow the primary running muscles to recover fast — even when increasing long run length
- Will also help most marathoners run faster in the marathon itself

Note: *You must still slow down the overall pace to at least 2 minutes per mile slower than you could currently run in a marathon.*

The most important walk breaks are the ones taken during the first mile and the second most important, those taken in the second mile, and so on. When taken from the beginning of all long runs, walk breaks erase fatigue, speed recovery, reduce injury, and yet bestow all of the endurance benefits of the distance covered. In other words, when both cover the same distance, a slow long run with walk breaks gives you the same distance conditioning as a fast run without them.

Doing "the minimum" will decrease your chance of injury and fatigue

The programs in this book might look minimal: only an hour of running during the week! But doing the minimum will decrease injury and fatigue. When you extend your endurance limits on each long run, you'll stress and break down the muscle and energy systems. The good news comes after rest days. When you give the running muscles a chance to recover, they make dozens of adaptations, gearing you up for an even greater challenge between one and three weeks later. If you're not getting enough rest, your muscles will accumulate pockets of microtears, which will continue to accumulate until you experience extreme fatigue or injury.

Tens of thousands of average people have gone through our program, with almost no injuries among those who follow the minimum. There are always some, however, who just have to push the envelope. The few who get injured in our training groups are almost always those who add distance, speed, or exercise days to our recommended schedule.

Because this is a bare-bones program, it's very important to do every one of the 50 minutes of exercise during the week to maintain long-run endurance and to speed recovery by increasing the blood flow to the muscles. You can run or walk in segments as short as 10 minutes, accumulating the magic 1 hour of exercise over a four- to five-day period. As is true with "cramming" before exams, it's not effective to get in all 60 minutes during the two days before the next long run. The day before the long run, avoid exercise, or at least avoid exercise for the calf muscles in the lower leg.

Rest and cross training

Significant rest is as important as the stress components of the program are. It's actually during the rest days that your muscles rebuild themselves, become stronger, and make adaptations for greater efficiency. Only if you refrain from stressing them will the muscles recover enough to prevent injury or lingering tiredness.

To maximize the chance of having resilient legs, you need to rest the muscles on the day before the long run. Cross training can be done on non-running days. Make sure that the lower leg muscles can recover and you don't seem to be accumulating overall fatigue. Avoid stair machines, leg-strengthening exercises, cycling that involves standing up, and step aerobics classes. *The most useful cross-training exercises are water running, cross-country ski machines, walking, swimming, cycling, and upper body weight training.*

Speed

Only those who have run a marathon before should even consider a time goal. The primary benefit in this program comes from gradually increasing the distance of the long run. Having run more than 60 marathons for time and more than 90 just to finish, I believe that time improvement is for the ego, although there's nothing wrong with that. The speed game can be interesting, but most of the satisfaction in running in a marathon comes from crossing the finish line. Your first marathon should be done at a pace slow enough so that you reach the finish line knowing that you could run faster and that you want to run another.

Veterans who have run a marathon or few and want to improve their times can add a speed component on some of the alternate ("off") weekends. *(See pp. 119–120*

for my recommended schedule of hill play.) Please be careful: The addition of speed will increase your chances of injury. As long as your goal is realistic, you're taking sufficient rest, and you adapt the pace to weather conditions, you'll give your body the creative stress it needs to help you improve gradually.

Veterans will increase their chance of fulfilling their time goals by increasing the length of the long run to 28 or 29 miles. This builds extra endurance, which gives your legs the capacity to keep pushing during the latter stages of the marathon itself. On these extra-long runs, reduce the pace from the beginning by running at least 2 minutes per mile slower than you could currently run in a marathon.

Don't mix and match

Beware of mixing components, that is, don't add speed-training elements to your long runs or try to extend or speed up the speed-training sessions. Running too fast on the long run will leave you much more tired, and with more damaged muscle cells, than you would experience by following the Two-Minute Rule. Not only are you increasing the chance of injury, but veterans who try to put speed into the endurance run will sacrifice the quantity or quality of their speed play later in the week. Often this fatigue is subtle, because of the release of stress hormones which mask the sensations of tiredness, and you won't feel it for two or three long runs.

Maintenance runs that are too fast will slow down recovery and increase the buildup of fatigue. It is important that your 60 minutes of maintenance exercise during the week is done slowly enough so the muscles will recover from the previous weekend. When in doubt, go slower.

Running too long or too fast during speed-play sessions will reduce the prospective benefit. In endurance events, speed, like endurance, is developed in a series of many speed sessions, each pushing only a little further than the one before. Going further or faster than you have been in the recent past will increase the time you need to recover and complicate the rebuilding process. When too many of the muscle cells are damaged, the muscle takes longer to rebuild itself.

It helps to have a group

One of the most delightful things I do is help set up training groups around North America. Each group member finds a significant motivation boost to do the long runs and to get in the 60 minutes during the week. You'll be inspired by your "teammates" some days, and you'll inspire them on others. Choose a team that has the same fitness condition as you. The goal is to go slowly enough on long runs that even the least-conditioned members of the group can keep up. In each of the cities where we have groups, we have several sub-groups, based upon fitness level.

FREQUENTLY ASKED QUESTIONS

Where is *the wall*?

Most marathoners who push themselves by starting their long runs too fast, or exceeding the distance of their current long run by more than 3 miles, or both, will experience a "wall" of fatigue at the end of the run. The wall hits you quickly as you reach your limits. Within a few meters, you go from feeling tired but capable of going on to feeling as if you can't go more than a few steps. The muscles have gone too far beyond their limit. Because of the physical stress, your left brain is sending you streams of messages that tell you to quit, question your sanity, and ask you philosophical questions such as, "Why am I doing this?"

Your wall is normally the length of your longest run within the past two or three weeks, provided you are running at the correct long-run pace. Going even a little too fast in the beginning will make you hit the wall sooner. On a hot, humid day —if you don't slow your pace down, way down—you'll bump into that wall before you know it. Even those who have missed a long run in their training schedule have been able to do the next long run by slowing down and running at least 3 minutes per mile slower than their current marathon pace, taking walk breaks much more frequently. The more conservative you are, in pace and in the number of walk breaks, from the beginning of the run, the more you can push your wall back farther and farther with little risk of fatigue or injury.

Why do I need to run a 26-mile training run before the marathon?

To prove to yourself that you can do it. On each long run, including the 26-miler, most people who are training for their first marathon are running farther than they have ever gone in their lives. After running the 26-mile training run, your training is complete. You won't have to push your wall back during the marathon itself. *You have arrived.*

The confidence bestowed by that 26-mile achievement will take away much of the nervousness leading up to the marathon itself. You're going to have some discouraging messages from that left side of the brain whenever you attempt a challenge like this, but you'll reduce them to a manageable level after completing this, the ultimate, long training run.

I've heard that going beyond 20 miles breaks you down. Is this true?

Only if you run too fast. Impatient runners and Type-A running personalities are the source of such rumors. They are so tired after an 18- to 20-mile run that they can't imagine how anyone could run longer than that without dire consequences. When long training runs themselves become races, the body accumulates fatigue, which may not be erased by marathon day.

It's an entirely different story when you follow the Two-Minute Rule and take the walk breaks you need. On each long run you gently push your endurance barrier back another 2 to 3 miles. Gentle fatigue, yes; breakdown, no.

> Yes, it's possible to complete every long one, even a 26-miler, without hitting the couch or bed for 12 hours.

But I have a time goal, even if it's my first run . . .

A time goal puts stress on you before and during the first marathon, which will reduce your enjoyment of the big moment. By backing off by two minutes per mile slower than your current marathon race pace, you'll be able to enjoy the course, talk to other runners and share the experience. You'll cross that finish line knowing that you could run faster, and this will motivate you to do just that . . . if you want to.

I ran my first 60 marathons hard. Now I've run more than 90 running within myself. I've received the same satisfaction, sense of achievement, and internal glow from all of the slow ones as I did from the fast ones. The main difference is that I could appreciate the satisfaction and celebrate the achievement on the slow ones. I wasn't very social for very long after the fast ones.

> Yes, it's possible to finish a marathon and celebrate with friends and family that evening.

Doesn't slow running produce a slow runner?

Actually, running a fast, long training run will make you run slower—your legs will be so dead they won't recover between the long runs. The long run has only one purpose: to build endurance. The most effective way to do this is progressively, by slowly covering 2 to 3 miles further than you covered on your previous long run. The slower you run, the more quickly you'll recover so that if you want to go for a fast time, you can do the speed training necessary to get faster.

What type of medical clearance do I need?

Before you start a strenuous training program, be sure to get clearance from a doctor who knows the benefits of exercise. Chances are slim that you'll have a problem that will prevent you from continuing, but let's make sure.

GALLOWAY'S PERFORMANCE PREDICTOR

Step 1: Run your "magic mile" time trial (MM). *(4 laps around the track)*

Step 2: *(Pace predicted is a very hard effort.)*

- **Half marathon predicted pace:** multiply MM by 1.2
- **Marathon predicted pace:** multiply MM by 1.3
- **10 Mile predicted pace:** multiply MM by 1.175

Example:

- **"Magic Mile" time:** 10:00
- **Marathon pace:** 10 × 1.3 = 13 minutes per mile
- **Half marathon pace:** 10 × 1.2 = 12 minutes per mile
- **10 Mile pace:** 10 × 1.175 = 11:45 minutes per mile
- **Long run training pace** = 15 minutes per mile
  (Add 2 minutes per mile to marathon pace regardless of goal distance.)

THE FIRST TIME I USED RUN-WALK-RUN: 1974

I opened my running store, Phidippides, in 1973 in a location that was not easy to find. The sales volume during the first few months was very slow, to put it nicely. I asked each customer for ideas about connecting with runners or prospective runners. One of the first customers worked in Florida State University's community lifestyle extension course department and suggested that I teach a class on "Beginning Running." I agreed.

During the first lesson, after each person described current conditioning and running history, I realized that this was, indeed, a group of novices. None had done any running for at least five years. So we started walking with a few one-minute jogs. On each jog, the group spread out a bit, which allowed me to set up groups based upon current running ability.

We divided into three groups. Young guys who played other sports formed the lead group. At the other end of the spectrum, about 10 members confessed that they had never exercised regularly, period. One of these folks described himself as a "basket case physical specimen" and the others embraced the name "basket cases." The middle group fell between the two.

I spent some time with each group, during the runs, to adjust the frequency of walk breaks so that no one was huffing and puffing—even at the end. Walk breaks kept the groups together. Everyone passed the final exam: finishing either a 5K or a 10K with smiles on their faces.

The best part for me was that there were no injuries. I had never been with a group of 20+ runners, at any time, who had run together for 10 weeks without any injuries.

I realized right away that the insertion of walk breaks was probably the single item that had kept my new runners out of the doctor's office. I've been using them ever since, continuing to fine-tune the ratios of running to walking based upon pace per mile (and individual needs). This has transformed the use of walk breaks into a method.

MY FIRST MARATHON

When I was 18 years old, in 1963, I entered the Atlanta Marathon. There were ten other starters. (Obviously marathons have gained a bit in popularity since those days!) I felt I could do pretty well, but there was one other runner I was worried about: Ken Wynn. Ken was 30 years old (ancient!) and a good road racer. I knew I could beat him on the track, but I didn't know about over such a long distance.

Ken was pretty casual: he pulled up in his car just before the start, and jumped out just as the gun went off. He left me in the dust, running about a 6-minute pace. I was doing about 7 minutes. I never saw him again.

The race was ten loops around Chastain Park. When I got to about 15 miles, I was pooped. The race director was on the course watching the runners, and I told him I was going to drop out. He said, "You can't, you're in first place!"

"What about Ken," I asked.

"He dropped out two laps ago."

Well all right, so on I went. I ran a few more laps, and felt awful. I came by the race director again and told him I wasn't feeling too good. This time he said "Are you sure you want to give up this trophy?" I'd never won a trophy before, so I went another lap. Now I was up to 20 miles and felt really bad.

Here was the director again. "Nothing you can say will keep me going here," I told him. He looked at his watch and said: "You're a half-hour ahead of second place."

OK, OK, that was enough incentive, so on I went. I ran and walked, struggling to the finish, and I won in 2:56:35.

It took me about two years before I felt like running another marathon. That experience kept playing over and over in my mind. Surely there's a better way of doing this, I thought, and it set me on the road to figuring out what I did wrong. How could this be done better, so it'd be easier, and you'd feel stronger without having to struggle so much? Through the years, it led me into developing the walk break strategy that's the central theme of this book.

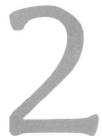

THE LONG RUN

"Since I've been running 26-milers in training, I don't hit the wall any more."

The long run is your marathon training program!

Whatever your goal, the long run will help you more than any component of your running program. By going slowly, you can burn more fat, push back your endurance barriers, and run faster at shorter distance races.

What is the long run?

The long run is your marathon training program. The long run, which, to begin with, you do once a week, is what builds up your endurance. At the outset, your long run is 3 miles. As you progress, you increase the distance by running further on each long run until you cover 10 miles. At that point, you'll run long every other weekend, increasing the distance by 2 miles each time. Once you reach 17 miles, you increase the distance by 3 miles every third week.

Building endurance

As you push a mile or three farther on each long run, you increase the limits of your endurance. It's important to go slowly on

---

THE MENTAL BENEFITS

There are significant and continuing physical benefits from doing long runs regularly, but the mental ones are greater. Each week, I hear from beginning marathoners after they have just run the longest run of their lives. They are excited, they've generated mental momentum, self-confidence, and a positive attitude.

---

each of these (follow the Two-Minute Rule) so your muscles can extend their current endurance limit. When it's really hot and humid, you'll need to run 2 or 3 minutes per mile slower. As you extend your long run to 26 miles, you build the exact endurance necessary to complete the marathon. (Those who have marathon time goals can extend their capacity by running as far as 30 miles for three to four weeks before the marathon.)

"When I got up to 10 miles and beyond, I started to feel some primitive feelings —like I was the first one blazing a trail for others to follow."

Walk breaks speed recovery

By walking early and often, you vary the use of the muscle and reduce the intensity of its work. Because you're not using the muscle in the same way continuously, you significantly increase the distance you can cover before fatigue sets in.

As the long runs get longer . . .

- Slow down the pace, from the beginning, by running at least two minutes per mile slower than your current marathon pace.
- Increase the frequency of walk breaks as the pace slows down.

Pacing of long runs: the Two-Minute Rule

Run all of the long runs at least two minutes per mile slower than predicted by the "magic mile." The walk breaks will help you to slow the pace, but you must run slower as well.

> You get the same endurance from the long run if you run slowly as you will if you run fast. However, you'll recover much faster from a slow long run.

Adjust for heat and humidity

The warmer and more humid it is, the slower you must go: 30 seconds per mile for every 5-degree increase above 60°F. More frequent walk breaks will also lessen the damage without detracting from the endurance benefits of that long run.

> **Hint:** Some runners bring thermometers or hand-held devices that can access current temperature.

SIGNS THAT YOU WENT TOO FAST ON A LONG RUN

- You need to hit the couch or bed and rest for an hour or more.
- Your muscles are sore or your legs fatigued for more than two days, and it becomes uncomfortable to run.
- Aches and/or pains last for more than four days.
- You huff and puff so much during the last 2 to 3 miles you can't carry on a conversation.
- You struggle during the last 2 to 3 miles to maintain pace or find yourself slowing down.
- You are nauseated and irritable at the end of the run.

Non-long-run weekends

On the non-long-run weekends, you have several options. Most runners will do a slow run of about half the distance of the current long run. On some of these "easy" weekends, it's wise to do a "magic mile" time trial to predict what you might be able to do in the marathon. Veterans will do speed sessions on some of the non-long-run weekends. If you're feeling good on these shorter runs, you can run them continuously, but there's no advantage in doing this. In other words, walk breaks are at your discretion on the shorter runs, including the ones during the week.

Almost everyone has at least one "bad" long run

You may never be able to discover why a long run may have been bad, but if you do know, learn from it! The tough ones teach you that you have hidden inner strengths, which you can draw upon in future challenges, both in running and in life itself. Knowing this will help your confidence and your ability to withstand adversity in the marathon itself.

> It doesn't hurt you to slow down on the long run, but you're going to have problems if you run faster than you should.

Faster recovery from long runs:

- Drink no more than 20 oz. of water per hour during a long run.
- Eat a snack within 30 minutes of completing the long run. The Endurox R4 sports drink supplies the 4:1 ratio of carbohydrates to protein which has been shown to speed recovery.
- Walk, while eating and drinking, for at least a mile.

- Soak your legs in a tub of cool water for 15 minutes. There must be a 20°F difference between body temperature and water temperature.

The death-defying warm-down

It's never a good idea to suddenly stop running and stand still. Several runners who had undiagnosed heart disease died when they finished a run and jumped immediately into the car or shower. Even if you have a very healthy heart, you'll speed up muscle recovery by gradually easing off the effort of the run.

- If it's an easy run, walk for 5–10 minutes before going to the car, shower, etc.
- At the end of a fast run, jog slowly for 5 minutes, walk and jog for 5 minutes, and then walk for 5 minutes.
- When you're racing, avoid the temptation to stop at the finish line. Jog for 5 more minutes and follow the rest of the recommendations for a fast run listed above.

LONG RUN FACTS:

- Twenty miles with walk breaks equals 20 miles run continuously . . . at any speed (but you recover faster with walk breaks).
- Forget about speed on long runs. Focus only on the component of endurance.
- *You can't run too slowly on the long runs.* Run at least 2 minutes per mile slower than the "magic mile" predicts in an all-out marathon, accounting for heat, humidity, etc.
- You won't usually feel bad when you're running too fast at the beginning of the run; you must force yourself to slow down.
- The day before the long run should be a no-exercise day.

3 THE GALLOWAY RUN-WALK-RUN METHOD

"Without walk breaks, I could run only 3 miles, with difficulty. Using walk breaks, I've finished three marathons feeling strong."

WALK BREAKS WILL...

- Allow those who can only run 2 miles to go 3 or 4 and feel fine
- Help beginners, heavy runners, or older runners to increase their endurance to 5K, 10K, or even the marathon in as little as six months
- Build up the endurance for runners of all abilities to go beyond "the wall"
- Allow runners over age 40 to not only do their first marathon but to improve times in most cases
- Help runners of all ages to improve times because legs are strong at the end
- Reduce the chance of injury and over-training to almost nothing

As one who has proudly run for more than five decades, I find it hard sometimes to admit this, but here goes. Our bodies weren't designed to run continuously for long distances, especially distances as long as the marathon. Sure we can adapt, but there is a better way to increase endurance than by running continuously. By alternating walking and running, from the start, there's virtually no limit to the distance you can cover. Thousands of people in their forties and fifties with no exercise background have used the run-walk-run method to train for, and complete a marathon after six months' training. Once we find the ideal ratio for a given distance,

walk breaks allow us to feel strong to the end and recover fast, while building up the same levels of stamina and conditioning that we would have reached if we had run continuously.

Most runners will record significantly faster times when they take walk breaks because they don't slow down at the end of a long run. Thousands of time-goal-oriented veterans have improved by 10, 20, 30 minutes and more in marathons by taking walk breaks early and often in their goal race. You can easily spot these folks in races. They're the ones who are picking up speed during the last 2 to 6 miles when everyone else is slowing down.

Our running heritage

Our ancient ancestors had to walk and run thousands of miles every year merely to survive. It is because they moved on to greener pastures and away from predators that we're here to philosophize about walk breaks. So it's a fact that each of us inherited an organism that was designed to move forward for long distances. As often happens with behaviors that promote survival, a series of complex and internally satisfying rewards has developed: the muscles relax, the creative and intuitive side of our brain is stimulated, and our spirits are energized. By getting out of the door and moving forward three or more times a week, even the most out-of-shape couch potato will discover this enhanced sense of self-worth and improved attitude.

Walking is our most efficient exercise pattern, but we can adapt to running and do well. Indeed, most walkers who add running to their exercise say they get a better boost in their after-exercise attitude. Running continuously, however, can quickly push us beyond the capacity of our leg muscles. When we alternate between walking and running, early and often, we are going back to the type of exertion that took our forebears across continents and over deserts and mountain ranges.

Walk breaks were part of the marathon — from the beginning

Ancient Greek messengers such as the original marathoner Phidippides regularly covered distances of more than 100 kilometers a day by walking and running. The accounts of the original marathon race, in the 1896 Olympics, described significant periods of walking for all competitors, including the winner Spiros Louis.

Elite marathoners continue to use walk breaks. The great American marathoner, Bill Rodgers, has said many times that he had to walk at water stations during his

EVEN A SHORT WALK BREAK WHEN TAKEN EARLY AND REGULARLY WILL:

- Restore resiliency to the main running muscles before they fatigue — like getting a muscle strength booster shot each break
- Extend the capacity of the running muscles at the end of the run because you're shifting the workload between the walking and the running muscles
- Virtually erase fatigue with each early walk break by keeping your pace and effort level conservative in the early stages
- Allow those with some types of previous injuries to knees, ankles, hips, feet, etc. to train for marathons without further injury
- Allow runners to improve 10 to 40 minutes in their marathon compared with running continuously
- Speed up recovery from each long run — even from 23- and 26-mile training runs
- Leave you feeling good enough to carry on social and family activities — even after the very long long runs

marathon victories in Boston and New York City in order to get the water into his stomach (instead of wearing it on his shirt). To conserve his resources, Fabian Roncero took several walk breaks during his victory in the Rotterdam Marathon in 1998. He finished in 2 hours, 7 minutes, and 26 seconds.

Running *faster* with walk breaks

Most runners will record significantly faster times when they take walk breaks because they don't slow down at the end of a long run. Thousands of veterans whose goal is to run faster have improved by 10, 20, 30 minutes and more in marathons by taking walk breaks early and often in the race. You can easily spot these folks: they're the ones who are picking up speed during the last 2 to 6 miles when everyone else is slowing down.

The title of marathoner has, from the beginning, been awarded to those who went the distance under their own power, whether they ran, walked, crawled, or tiptoed. When you cross that finish line, you've joined an elite group. About one-tenth of 1 percent of the population does this each year. Don't let anyone take that great achievement away from you.

I've now done well over 150 marathons, about half of them without walk breaks. On every one of the walk-break marathons, I received the same sense of accomplishment, all of the internal rewards, and the indescribable exhilaration of finishing as on the non-walk-break marathons. But when I inserted walk breaks throughout, I was able to enjoy the accomplishment afterward.

> "When I moved my weekend long run up to 10 miles, I started to feel, after each long run, some primitive feelings—like I was the first one blazing a trail for others to follow."

Why do walk breaks work?

> By using muscles in different ways—from the beginning—your legs keep their bounce as they conserve resources.

By varying the use of your muscles, your legs keep their bounce as they conserve resources. Walk breaks keep you from using up your resources early. By alternating the exertion level and the way you're using your running muscles, these prime movers have a chance to recover before they accumulate fatigue. On each successive walk, most or all of the fatigue is erased, giving you strength at the end. This dramatically reduces damage to the muscles, allowing you to carry on your life activities even after a marathon.

Walk breaks force you to slow down early in the run so that you don't start too fast. This conserves your energy, fluids, and muscle capacity. On each walk break, the running muscles make internal adaptations, which give you the option to finish under control, increase the pace, or go even further. When a muscle group, such as your calf, is used continuously step after step, it tires relatively soon. The weak areas get overused and force you to slow down later or scream at you in pain afterward. By shifting back and forth between walking and running muscles, you distribute the workload among a variety of muscles and increase your overall performance capacity. For veteran marathoners, this is often the difference between achieving a time goal or not.

Walk breaks can eliminate injury

> "I tried to train for three marathons without walk breaks and became injured each time. Walk breaks allowed me to get to the starting line and then to the marathon finish line . . . injury free!"

Many runners who were injured during previous training programs (because they ran continuously) have stayed injury-free when they added walk breaks to long runs. If you don't walk from the beginning, your leg muscles fatigue more quickly and can't keep those lower extremities moving efficiently in their proper range of motion. The resulting wobble allows the leg to extend too far forward in an over-stride. This abuses the tendons and injures the small muscle groups that try to keep the body on its proper mechanical track but don't have the horsepower to control the body weight moving forward.

Walk breaks taken early in the run keep the muscles strong and resilient enough so that the legs can move with strength and efficiency throughout. This will significantly reduce or eliminate the excess stress around the knees, ankles, feet, etc. that produces injury. The little "back-up" muscle groups can stay in reserve and fine-tune the running motion after fatigue sets in.

> Walk breaks can change a bad run into a regular one and sometimes a great one.

When to take walk breaks

The earlier you take the walk breaks, the more they help you! To receive maximum benefit, you must start the walk breaks in the first mile, before you feel any fatigue. If you wait until you feel the need for a walk break, you've already reduced your potential performance. Even waiting until the 2-mile mark to take the first break will reduce the resilience you could regain from walking in the first mile. To put it in shopping terms, would you like a discount? Walk breaks earn you a discount from the pounding on legs and feet. If you walk often enough, start early enough, and keep the pace slow enough, a 10-mile run leaves you no more tired than if you had run only 5 to 7 miles and a 20-miler makes you only as tired as a 12- to 15-mile run would.

Walk breaks can change a bad run into a regular one — and sometimes a into a great one. Sometimes we may not feel good as we start a run. Instead of quitting or suffering through (and then not wanting to run the next time), try a 1-minute walk break every 1 to 5 minutes. By breaking up your run early and often, you can still cover the distance you'd like to cover on that day, burn the calories you'd like to burn, and increase the chance that you'll enjoy the experience of running itself.

You don't need to take walk breaks on runs that are short enough and easy for you to run continuously. For example, if your Tuesday run is 3 miles and you feel good, you don't need to put in walk breaks. If the walk breaks can make the experience better, however, take them!

> "I waited until the 10-mile mark to take walk breaks in my first two marathons—and was wiped out for two weeks. When I took them every mile, from the beginning, I improved my time by 20 minutes, recovered fast, and danced afterwards."

PASS THE BUCK

If you feel wimpy about walking early, carry an empty water bottle and pretend to drink as you walk. You can also blame me: Tell those who pass you that Jeff Galloway made you do it!

When in doubt, walk

It's much better to take a 1-minute walk break every 5 minutes than to take a 5-minute walk every 25 minutes. By breaking up your run early—with even a short break—you allow for quicker and more effective recovery. If you're used to walking for 1 minute every 4 minutes but are not feeling good at the beginning of a run, walk for 1 minute after running for 2, or for 30 seconds after running for 1 minute.

There's very little difference in benefit between these two intervals, but the more frequent break (a 30-second walk after a 1-minute run) will keep the legs fresher. The longer you run continuously, the more fatigued the legs become. Remember that you lose only about 13 seconds when you walk for 1 minute. The short distance you lose on extra walking earlier will almost always be recovered at the end—because

you kept your legs fresh. Those who put this concept to the test almost always find that taking more frequent walk breaks doesn't slow the overall time of long runs—when the long runs are done at the correct slow pace.

How fast should I walk?

A slow walk is fine. When walking fast for 1 minute, most runners will lose about 10–12 seconds over running at their regular pace. But, even if you walk slowly, you'll lose only about 17–20 seconds. If you have a Type-A running personality and want to walk fast, make sure that you don't lengthen your walking stride too much. Monitor the tightness of your hamstrings and the tendons behind the knee. If you feel tension there, walk slowly with bent knees to keep that area relaxed. A slow walk is just as good as a fast one and may keep the leg muscles from getting tight.

Racewalking technique is not recommended, but a shorter stride with quick turnover is OK when practiced regularly.

How often should I walk?

Even if you run the same distance every day, you'll find that you'll need to vary the frequency of your walk breaks to account for speed, hills, heat, humidity, time off from training, etc. If you expect that your run will be more difficult or will require a longer recovery, take more frequent walk breaks (or longer walks); you may be surprised at how quickly you recover. On cold days, you may not need to take the walks as often (although it's not wise to reduce walk breaks in any run longer than 17 miles).

Can walk breaks make me run faster?

Surveys of veteran marathoners have shown an average improvement of over 13 minutes when they put walk breaks into their marathon, rather than running continuously under the same conditions. By conserving the strength and efficiency of the running muscles through early walk breaks, you'll avoid the slowdown in the last 6 miles, where most continuous runners lose their momentum. By making sure to walk before you get tired, you will be able to run with strength to the finish line, avoiding the 7- to 15-minute slowdown at the end. With proper speed training, pacing, and the right ratio of walking to running, you'll run faster during the last 6 to 8 miles because you walked early.

I've heard from over 100 runners who've broken 3 hours in the marathon for the first time after inserting a walk break every mile.

The mental benefit: Breaking 26 miles into segments which you know you can do

Even runners who can finish a marathon in less than 3 hours continue to take their walk breaks to the end. One of them explained it this way: "Instead of thinking at 20 miles that I had 6 more gut-wrenching miles to go, I was saying to myself, 'One more mile until my break.' Even when it was tough, I always felt that I could go 1 more mile." Another marathoner who uses a 3-minute run and a 1-minute walk regime told me that she got over the tough parts by saying, "Three more minutes."

A game of "chase"

Another mental trick is to turn the marathon into a game of chase. After a few miles into your marathon, you'll settle into a pace and notice some of the folks around you. As you take your walk break, track one or two of them so that you catch up with them by the time you start your next walk break. You'll have to pick new markers around the halfway point. Because they're running continuously, your original "hares" will probably start slowing down about then.

Walk breaks in the marathon: How long and how often?

The following regime is recommended for the first 18 miles of the marathon. After that, walk breaks can be reduced or eliminated as desired.

First-time marathon runners Follow the program you used in your last long run as long as you finished strong and recovered fast. If you struggled during the last few miles, take walk breaks more often from the beginning. Use the Run-Walk-Run Strategy table below.

Those whose long run is 20 miles or less There's still hope. Let's say that you picked up this book less than three weeks before your marathon and your longest run is only 18 miles, but you had no trouble with your last long run and have been taking walk breaks. In the marathon add 1 minute per mile to your projected finish pace and use the Run-Walk-Run Strategy table on the next page. For example:

Projected marathon pace: 9:00
But long run was only 18 miles.
So new marathon pace is 10:00.
Run-walk-run strategy is 3–1.

Run-Walk-Run Ratios for runners

Here are my recommended ratios of running and walking, based upon your pace per mile. These ratios are in effect for both training runs and during the marathon itself.

Runners: Remember that long runs should be at least 2 minutes per mile slower than your projected finish pace in the full marathon. An additional slowdown should be made for increased temperature: 30 seconds per mile slower for each 5 degrees of temperature increase above 60°F. It is always safer to take more frequent breaks.

Walkers: Shuffle for 30 seconds after 2 to 4 minutes of regular walking—from the beginning.

Run-Walk-Run Strategy

Training Pace	Run	Walk
7 minutes per mile	1 mile	30 seconds
8 minutes per mile	4 minutes	30 seconds
9 minutes per mile	4 minutes	1 minute
10 minutes per mile	3 minutes	1 minute
11 minutes per mile	2½ minutes	1 minute
12 minutes per mile	2 minutes	1 minute
13 minutes per mile	1 minutes	1 minute
14 minutes per mile	30 seconds	30 seconds
15 minutes per mile	30 seconds	45 seconds
16 minutes per mile	30 seconds	60 seconds
17 minutes per mile	20 seconds	60 seconds
18 minutes per mile	15 seconds	60 seconds
19 minutes per mile	10 seconds	45 seconds
20 minutes per mile	5–10 seconds	60 seconds

Walk Break Questions

Do I need to take walk breaks on the short runs during the week?

If you can now run continuously on shorter midweek runs, you don't have to take the walk breaks. If you want to take them, do so. Walk breaks on midweek runs will insure that you recover from the long runs as quickly as possible.

Do I have to take walk breaks at the end of my runs if my legs are tightening up?

Take walk breaks as long as you can because they will speed your recovery. If your legs cramp up later during walk breaks then just shuffle through the breaks (by keeping your feet low to the ground and taking a short stride). At the end of a run, you want to stay as fluid as you can while still alternating the use of the muscle groups. Cramping at the end tells you to start more slowly with more frequent walk breaks in the next long run and to avoid dehydration the day before the run, the morning of the run, and during the run itself.

Should I change my run/walk ratio during the marathon?

If you're feeling good at the 13- to 15-mile point, you could stretch the running segments by 1 additional minute: instead of running for 4 minutes and walking for 1 minute (9 minute-per-mile pace), you could run for 5 minutes and walk for 1 minute. After 18 miles, you could keep same regime and add another minute of running, or omit the walk breaks entirely. Most marathoners who are feeling good still take at least a 30-second break every mile. If, however, you're having a bad day, increase the frequency of walk breaks or walk more slowly during each break, and you'll be less likely to slow down at the end of the marathon.

If I've never tried the walk breaks in training runs, would you advise my taking them in the marathon?

Walk breaks will only help you. I've received hundreds of letters, faxes, e-mails, and calls from those who heard about the walk break concept the evening before a marathon and tried it the next day. Their response is very similar to this one.

Can I benefit from a walk break even though my time goal is under three hours?

Yes. More than 100 runners have reported breaking 3 hours by taking walk breaks when they couldn't do so by running continuously.

A growing number of runners have run below 2:50 by taking walk breaks at least during the first 18 miles. Everyone benefits from walk breaks. They reduce the pounding, allow you to drink enough water, and speed up recovery from long runs. Competitive runners can erase enough fatigue during the first half so that they can race the second half. The demands of a time-goal program require quick recovery, which walk breaks allow. By following the Two-Minute Rule and taking liberal walk breaks from the beginning, you can be recovered enough from a 26- to 28-mile run to do speed training within two to four days.

ARE WALK BREAKS FOR WIMPS?

A friend of mine in his late forties had been trying for years to run a 3:30 marathon, but 3:40 was as fast as he could run. According to the times of his 5K and 10K races, he should have been able to finish in about 3:25. He had done plenty of intense training in three different marathon campaigns, including high mileage, lots of speedwork, two runs a day, etc. Eventually, I told him that if he didn't run below 3:30 in his goal marathon, I'd return his check, and he sent in his entry form for my program. I never mentioned the walk breaks because I knew he would say something about "sissy stuff" and not sign up. I also knew that in the past he had probably over-trained for his goal and mainly needed to run with a group to slow down his pace on the long run.

After the very first session he came up to me, irate, and demanded his money back. "I can't do these walk breaks: they're wimpy!" I refused to return his check, reminding him that a deal was a deal. So he completed the program, complaining during just about every walk break. Secretly, he told friends in his pace group, he wasn't going to walk during the marathon itself.

On marathon morning, his group leader lined up with him and physically restrained him for 1 minute each mile, making him walk. Then, at 18 miles, the leader looked at my friend and said, "Well, you seem to have just enough life in your legs, so run along now!" And he did. His time was 3:25. He had run that marathon 15 minutes faster than ever before!

At first, he couldn't believe that he could improve that much while walking every mile. But when he analyzed his past marathons, he found that he had always slowed down in the last 6 to 8 miles. In this marathon, he kept picking up the pace after those first 18 miles and had knocked 5 minutes off his time in the last segment. He was forced to admit that the early and regular muscle shifts left his legs feeling strong and responsive all the way to the finish line.

"When I heard you recommend walk breaks at the seminar before the marathon, I didn't want to think about it. I don't know why but it just seemed demeaning for a real runner like me to walk like that. You see, I've run ten marathons with a personal best of 3:57 and have been proud of the fact that I've never walked.

"But after thinking about it overnight, I decided to prove you wrong by doing exactly what you suggested. To tell you the honest truth, I'd been sick for the last couple of weeks or so and calculated that I probably couldn't run a personal best anyway.

"I walked for a minute every mile and, during the running portions, ran my original goal pace for a 3:55 finish.

"By the first half of the marathon I was behind my goal pace by 3 minutes. Aha, I said to myself, Galloway is going to be wrong. If I'm already 3 minutes behind at the half, I'll be way behind at the finish.

"At 20 miles, I was beginning to feel stronger than I had ever felt at that stage of the marathon. I cut out the walk breaks and ran to the finish, except for short breaks at water stops. Although tired during the last 6 miles, I felt good and passed a lot of people, not really aware of my pace.

"I couldn't believe my time at the finish: 3:52 — 5 minutes faster than I had ever run in my life . . . and after a bad cold! How did that happen?"

"My first exposure to the Galloway Program was at the 1999 Disney World Marathon, where a Runner's World Pace Leader lead a group to a sub-3:30 finish. It was a 4-minute PR for me, my first Boston qualifier, and the most comfortable finish of seven marathons. Realizing the dream of running Boston wouldn't have been possible without the 'walk break.'"

4 RUNNING FORM

> Marathon form is most efficient when you don't feel as if you are making any noticeable effort.

If it ain't broke . . .

Running form is most efficient when you're cruising along, almost on automatic. Over several years, your running form becomes more efficient—even if you still feel clunky. In fact, when runners change their form in an attempt to run better, they have often been forced to do so because they have been injured or excessively fatigued due to bad form. Even so, it's almost always better to go with the natural flow of your legs and body—even if you don't look like a star. In other words, *if nothing seems to be wrong with your form, don't try to fix it.* But if you're experiencing some of the form-related problems noted at the end of this chapter, I have a prescription for moving more easily.

Distance running does not require strength. Instead of overcoming gravity, we're trying to minimize its effect by staying low to the ground and reducing extraneous body motion. By going slowly in the beginning, it's easy to get moving, and, once in motion, the body wants to stay in motion. I use three components to monitor and fine-tune running form: **posture**, **bounce**, and **over-stride**.

Posture

Don't try to be a Marine at attention. The best posture for running, walking, or cruising is just good posture, with all elements relaxed and balanced as the foot comes underneath. A forward lean forces you to shorten your stride and creates extra tension on the lower back and neck. A backward lean is unusual but will also produce a shorter stride, loss of power from the running stride, and possible tension in the lower back.

Some will argue that a forward lean will help you run faster, but I've found this to help only for a hundred meters or so. It forces you to work harder and therefore spend resources that are then not available later in the run and you lose more time than you gained during the short burst. The only exception I've found to this rule is when running on a gradual, downhill grade. A slight forward lean can help you run faster, and the boost from downhill gravity will offset the decrease in stride length. A forward lean is often the cause of lower back pain or neck pain.

Like a puppet on a string

To correct forward lean, create a mental image (during the form drill) of yourself suspended from the very top of your head by a giant string as if you were a puppet. The effect is to lift you upright—head in line with shoulders and hips and everything lined up with each foot as it assumes the body's weight. The image also helps you to stay light on your feet.

The first effect of being a good puppet is to have your body line up without any tension—you're in balance. Walk around with the image of the puppet on the string until you feel relaxed in this upright position. Then start running slowly. On your days for form work, you may then accelerate for between 50 and 150 meters, running as a lightly balanced puppet. Not only does the posture correct itself, but also your chest is forward as are your hips, allowing for a quick touch-off with the feet. You may have to make little adjustments, but when you are aligned in a relaxed mode, running will be easier and you'll feel less effort in the legs.

Bounce

When in doubt, use less energy and stay lower to the ground, and you'll run faster, more smoothly, and with better leg turn-over. The energy spent in bouncing too high even by an inch is wasted—burned up in the air. The higher you lift yourself off the ground, the greater the shock you have to absorb when landing and the longer it'll take for your feet and legs to recover from that run. Excess bounce also forces the legs to go through inefficient, extraneous motion during the extra time in the air. A higher back kick, for example, is the result of excess leg swing because your body is off the ground for an extra second or so. Such a kick produces early fatigue in the hamstring muscles.

> The feet should not spring dramatically off the ground.

You can correct bounce by keeping your feet close to the ground during sections of every run, especially when you feel the temptation to bounce, which is usually during the first mile and when going downhill. Instead of bouncing and spending energy, save your resources with a quick and light lift-off of the foot. You'll run about as fast by staying low to the ground and taking more steps per minute.

> Stay light on your feet.

Over-stride

As the forward leg absorbs body weight, the lower part should not be extended out in front of you. The tendency to over-stride is another attempt to counter slowing down with a quick fix. Unfortunately, our intuitive sense of pace gets us into trouble here. As runners get tired and realize that the main driving muscles are weakening because of fatigue, they subconsciously lengthen their stride to speed themselves up. This is another quick fix that will help for a short distance but is counterproductive later.

Longer strides will over-stretch the muscles, causing them to tighten up later and weaken. Too long a stride can put the knees or the muscles out of efficient mechanical range, increasing recovery time and causing injury. Everybody has weak links, places that tend to get injured most often. When the main driving muscles are tired, the knees wobble more and the weak links are likely to be pushed beyond their capacity.

> Feet should stay low to the ground.

Shorten your stride

When you feel tension in muscles that are at their limits—especially the calf and hamstring groups—you need to shorten the stride a bit to relax them. Keep on shortening your stride until the leg muscles do relax. This may allow you to pick up the turnover of the feet and legs. But even if this increase doesn't happen, you'll reduce the chance of injury caused by the increased fatigue of over-striding and speed up recovery. Often, the only adjustment needed is a shortening of an inch or two, but the relaxation it provides will allow the legs to go at a faster rhythm. Some runners can actually speed up at the end of the race.

As you pick up the turnover on form accelerations, be sure to keep the stride short enough so the leg muscles are relaxed and maintain a quick rhythm. When in doubt, keep the stride short so you can maintain a light, quick step on each of these pick-ups.

Turnover Drill

As runners become faster, their stride length decreases. Therefore, the way to get faster is to increase the turnover of feet and legs. Even those who lack a fast bone in their bodies will benefit from turnover drills because they teach the body to find a more efficient motion.

THE DRILL

After a slow 1-mile warm-up, select a level and traffic-free stretch of road, trail, or track. Without picking up your speed, count the number of times either your left foot or your right comes down in 30 seconds. Jog or walk for a minute or so and then run back, counting again for 30 seconds, with the goal of increasing the count by one or two. Repeat this four to six times, with the same projected increase each time but without a significant increase in effort.

If you do this drill once a week, you'll intuitively learn to stay low to the ground with an increasingly lighter touch of the foot. If you do this drill at least once a week, a year from now you'll be running faster and with no increase in effort. The increased turnover and improved efficiency also makes running feel easier. You'll see more progress if you do it twice a week. But you'll lose two weeks of progress if you miss a week.

Troubleshooting form problems
Quads

When the main running muscles get tired, your stride shortens as you slow down. The best strategy in this situation is to shorten the stride a little more and allow for a slight slowdown. Many runners will, however, try to maintain the same pace by using other muscles. The quadriceps on the front of your leg above the knee can permit you to do this for a while by lifting the leg and maintaining the longer stride length. But the quads are not designed for this and they tire easily. Afterward, you can usually count on at least two to four days of soreness.

Sometimes soreness in the quads is directly related to more downhill running than you are used to. Even when using a short stride while running downhill, some effort is required of the quadriceps muscles —especially on long hills. Many runners aggravate this by over-striding as they go down. Yes, it is tempting, and it is easy to extend the lower leg out in front of the body too much to pick up speed. To keep the legs and body under control, the quads must then be used as brakes. Not only is this an inefficient use of muscle power, but also your quads will complain for several days afterward, especially after a long run. The recommended technique is to maintain a short stride and let gravity move you down with little effort.

Light exercise every day (such as walking on flat terrain) will speed up the recovery of sore quads. It's not a good idea to massage them, stretch them, or exercise them too hard while they are sore.

Behind the knee

Another sign of over-striding is pain or increased discomfort behind the knee. When you reach out further than you should with the lower leg, you move out of the knee's efficient range of motion. The full impact of your body's weight must be supported by the knee and through a mechanical range in which it is weakened. This is a hinge joint and was designed only

to support body weight in the act of moving forward, with the foot directly underneath.

When your main running muscles become tired, they cannot give the knee any protection from this repeated abuse. As the tendons behind the knee become more stretched out during the run, the knee is forced to support the weight of the body in a straight or locked out position. Downhill running and faster running tend to bring on this problem.

Always try to maintain some bend in each knee when running. A shorter stride length will reduce the chance of this over-stride problem. Do not try to stretch the tendons behind the knee at any time. Light massage with a chunk of ice can help. (Get a doctor's permission before using anti-inflammatory drugs.)

Wobbly running form

Most runners feel great at the beginning of long runs. It's natural to be tired at the end, but when the legs aren't supporting you well, you've overdone it in the beginning. The danger of this condition is that you can easily aggravate your weak links, those areas in which you tend to experience injury.

The condition is entirely preventable. Start the long runs a lot more slowly—at a pace that is at least 2 minutes slower per mile than you could run a marathon on that day. It is also wise to take 1-minute walk breaks every 1–3 minutes from the beginning!

Shoulder and neck muscles

If you're leaning forward as you run, you'll have a tendency to compensate by holding the head back, which uses the muscles of the shoulder and neck more and produces fatigue more rapidly. When the body is held upright, the head, neck, and shoulders are in alignment and require little or no muscle power to keep them in position.

Those who hold their arms too far out from the body will also overextend the muscles of the shoulder and neck. The ideal arm motion is minimal, with the arms held in a relaxed position next to the body. When the lower arm goes through a small range of motion alongside the shorts and the upper part of the arm hardly moves, there is little fatigue in the arms, shoulders, or neck muscles.

Lower back

Another sign of too much forward lean is a tired and tight lower back. By maintaining an upright body posture, you'll avoid the tendency to overstress the back. If you think that your back muscles are weaker than they should be, talk to a physical therapist about some strength exercises to compensate. One which has worked well for me is "arm running." Do not try this or any strength exercise, however, until you've been given clearance by a strength expert. *(See p. 33.)*

Hamstrings

If your hamstrings are sore, you are lifting the foot behind you too far and/or extending your stride too much. The longer stride is particularly a problem at the end of the long run as it overextends muscles, such as the hamstring, that are already tight and tired. Try to keep your stride short, especially at the end of the run. In your back leg motion the lower part of the leg should —at its highest elevation—be parallel to the horizontal.

Knee pain

When the main driving muscles get tired, they can no longer control your safe range of motion, and the resulting wobble can leave you in pain, sore, or injured. A slower early pace, and walk breaks, will help the legs stay fresh.

Sore feet and lower legs

You're pushing off the ground too hard and probably too high. Stay closer to the ground, touching it lightly, and maintain a short stride.

For more information on running form, see *Galloway's Book on Running*.

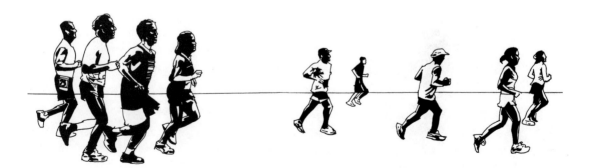

EFFICIENCY WINS

A classic confrontation occurred in 1995 in the Boston Marathon between the efficiency of a marathoner and the strength and power of a 5K–10K runner. From the starting gun, Uta Pippig looked as if she were cutting her classic marathoner's stride too short. Her closest competitor, Elena Meyer, appeared to be playing her cards right by going out slowly, forcing Uta to shoulder all of the pressure of setting the pace.

By the midpoint, Uta had built a modest lead and was running so smoothly that her quick turnover gave the appearance of weakness. With a tiny stride and no knee lift, she appeared to be jogging. This signaled to several experienced observers that it just wasn't her day. Elena sensed this and began her drive to overtake the leader. The South African's strong, athletic leg motion led many experts to say that it was only a matter of time before she would pull even with the German.

At 15, 17, and 19 miles, it continued to appear that Meyer's long and powerful stride must be taking big chunks out of Pippig's lead. The TV commentators noted how wimpy the German's turnover appeared. But to the surprise of all, a time check showed that Pippig's lead was *increasing* slightly.

By 22 miles, Meyer had dropped out with muscle cramps and Pippig had picked up her pace. But on camera, she still looked like a jogger. That short and wimpy stride with no knee lift resulted in a 2:26 marathon—one of the fastest woman's times of the year.

5 CROSS TRAINING

On non-running days, cross training (XT) can give the attitude boost we need while it bestows additional conditioning. The best programs are those that are fun and therefore draw you back to do them again and again. For this reason, many marathon runners do a variety of exercises in a single cross-training session to reduce the chance of boredom and burnout. Cross training is also used to maintain marathon conditioning while runners are recovering from injury. With cross training, you don't have to think that it's over if you come down with an injury during a marathon program. Over the years, I've met dozens of runners who, although injured, maintained their conditioning through significant cross training and were able to finish the marathon comfortably. During an eight-week injury, one runner ran in the water and came back to do the marathon in a personal best: under 3 hours!

The best exercises

As in any form of conditioning, the best exercises to use as back-ups for the running muscles are those that best use the leg muscles as they are used in running. Water running has produced the best effect for large numbers of marathoners. Cross-country ski machines have also produced a high level of running conditioning. For burning fat, the best exercises are those that elevate the body temperature, keep it up, and use lots of muscle cells. Cross-country ski machines, rowing machines, cycling and other indoor machines can help to increase the fat-burning effect.

Because stair machines use many of the muscles that are used in running they aren't the best choice for alternative exercise on a rest day from running. But they can simulate hill running, to some extent, if you use them occasionally to replace a running day (or as a second running session on a running day).

CROSS-TRAINING SCHEDULE

Mon	Tue	Wed	Thu	Fri	Sat	Sun
Water run	Cycle	Water run	Swim	Water run	Off	Long water run
Weight training	Swim	Strength training	Cross-country ski machine	Strength training	Swim	

Easing into new exercises

- On the first day go 5 easy minutes, rest for 20 to 30 minutes, and then go for 5 more minutes.

- You could start with two to three different exercises, alternating them and gradually increasing the session to 1 hour. To get the best effect for the marathon, it's better to use a slow continuous motion instead of quick, short bursts of high intensity.

- During each successive session, increase each of the two segments by 3 to 5 minutes.

CROSS-TRAINING INCREMENTS

Session No.	Exercise A	Exercise B
	(minutes)	
1	5	5
2	8	8
3	12	12
4	15	15
5	18	18
6	22	22

- Build up to about the same duration and intensity of exercise you'd be doing if running.

- Exercise every day at first, if you wish, building up to two 30-minute sessions. You may then combine the exercise into one continuous session every other day. On the days between, you may do a different exercise routine. *(See, for example, the schedule on p. 29.)*

- In individual exercises or in the session as a whole, never push the muscles to the point of tiredness or loss of strength.

If you have been injured, don't do any exercise that could aggravate the injury. Plan your cross-training exercise to simulate the intensity and duration of your scheduled running session for that day. For example, if a long run is scheduled, estimate the length of the time you'd be running and spend that time continuously running in the water, on the cross-country ski machine, and so on. As you're doing the alternative exercise, try to maintain about the same level of exertion as you would when running.

WATER RUNNING
Benefits

- Because the legs must find the most efficient mechanical path through the water, extraneous motions of the feet and legs are reduced or eliminated over time.

- The water's resistance strengthens muscles that can provide back-up strength to the primary running muscles. By alternating off and on, the main running muscles will retain their resilience longer. The smaller reserve muscles will also be able to keep you going for a little while if you overuse the main running muscles and need some help to keep running during the last few miles in the marathon.

- You get a great cardiovascular training session without any pounding. Because the prime running muscles are not being used, most injuries can heal.

Techniques

The marathon motion

Use the same running form in the water that you would use when running efficiently on land. The body should be upright, not stiff. A slight forward lean is okay, but don't lean too far. The ideal motion is a smooth one, getting quick turnover. Focus on finding the most efficient path through the water. In this way you'll be cutting out mechanical inefficiencies and encouraging an efficient stride on land.

- Knees don't come up very far.
- Lower legs and feet are kicked forward.
- The whole leg is brought behind you, with the knee slightly bent.
- The back leg bends to a right angle and then returns forward.
- Arms can be moved through a range of motion similar to that of regular running. Don't exaggerate the arm-swing.

Cross-country ski motion

A strengthening exercise, the cross-country ski motion should be done in short segments of between 10 seconds and 1 minute. By weaving segments into the marathon motion, you'll increase strength in the quadriceps (front of thigh), hamstrings, butt muscles, hip flexors, and lower back.

- The legs are almost completely straight.
- The range of motion is about 20 percent longer than the range of the marathon motion.
- Move the legs like scissors through the water.

Start each segment with a short range of motion and extend it gradually. Over time, you may increase both range of motion and speed, but be careful. Remember that you're building strength and not anaerobic performance. Never extend any motion to the point that you feel you have reached your mechanical limits. And don't work so long that you're out of breath.

Sprinting

For those who have been doing speed play and don't want to risk injury while in a marathon program, the sprint motion can keep the speed components in good form without the risk of pounding or incurring interval-training injuries.

- Shorten your marathon motion to about half.
- Keep legs and feet directly underneath you.
- Pick up the turnover of your legs and feet so that you're going through the leg pattern about twice as fast as you go through the marathon motion.

This shouldn't be a true sprint (going all out) because you want to go at a pace that you could continue for 1 to 2 minutes. You will be huffing and puffing through the second half of each of these, as they are anaerobic. Start each sprint segment by gradually increasing the turnover. The short range of motion directly underneath you will cause your head and shoulders to rise out of the water somewhat. To keep up with the legs, the arm motion should also be a shortened version of the marathon motion.

Precautions

- Make sure that the water running motion is within efficient mechanical range.
- If you're injured, get clearance from your doctor to make sure that you're not aggravating the injury.
- Don't over-train. Just going through an efficient water running motion will bestow benefits. No need to push it.

STRENGTH TRAINING

I don't believe that we need to do any strength exercises to run a marathon. If you have any doubts, look at the "toothpick" limbs of the winners of any major marathon. It's obvious that they don't spend time in the gym. The most important physics concept for running, in my opinion, is inertia. Running is easier and more fun when we spend a little energy to get moving and then fine-tune our movements to take advantage of our momentum.

I do, however, recommend a couple of strength exercises for long-term postural support. Strong and balanced postural muscles will keep you upright when you're fatigued, and improve your breathing and oxygen intake enabling you to maintain running strength and efficiency. I discovered this after my arms and shoulders were getting increasingly tired on long runs in the mid-1980s. By doing the exercises listed below, I've virtually eliminated that type of fatigue — even in marathons.

Leg strength

Legs can be strengthened most efficiently by doing regular hill training *(see pp. 117–121)*. Running up an incline forces the leg muscles to perform against natural resistance. By doing artificial weight exercises, you can upset the natural balance that has developed between the muscle groups. Such an imbalance can cause injury. If you want to develop strength, it helps to see a strength expert. The exercises I am suggesting are those that work for me as a runner.

Postural strength exercises

I've found that a bare minimum of strength training can keep the postural muscles strong and balanced. These muscles maintain the upper body in a relaxed but upright position. When neglected, they slowly weaken. Over a ten-year period, individuals gradually slump and stoop a little more. Runners notice this sooner. On long or hard runs, those with weak postural muscles will lose their form more quickly, their pace will slow, and recovery time will increase. A slumping upper body also cuts down on the efficiency of breathing and reduces oxygen absorption. After starting with about ten exercises in the late 1980s, I gradually refined them to the two that are described below. The **crunch** strengthens the front of the body, and **arm running** strengthens the muscles of the lower back, upper back, shoulders, and neck. If you're looking for beach muscles, this isn't the right program!

Crunches

This is the old sit-up with the range of motion reduced significantly. By keeping the body near the floor and constantly using the muscles, you get a lot of good strengthening in a short time. This exercises the upper abdominal group (the "six-pack").

1. Lie down on a padded surface on your back and with your *knees bent.*

2. Raise your upper torso very slightly off the floor; the lower back should still be touching the surface. Lift and lower no more than 3 to 5 inches or so and repeat until the muscles are tired.

Don't continue until the muscles give out.

Arm running

This exercise is done in the standing position with legs spread about as wide as your shoulders. You can experiment a little bit with the motion, but don't do anything that will put your back at risk. It's always safer, when using handheld weights, to keep them close to the body.

1. Stand upright and relaxed with your feet spread about the width of your shoulders or closer if shoulder-width is not comfortable.

2. Use handheld weights in both hands, choosing a weight that will give you a little challenge but is not a struggle.

3. Move the arms through the motion you'd use when running, keeping the hands close to the body.

4. Starting with two or three repetitions, increase by one rep each session until you get up to ten.

To see results, you need to do this twice or three times a week. I do several sets of ten, spread throughout the day, for three days a week.

> "Thanks to the Galloway Program this is the first year that I've been able to stick to my long run schedule and go into a big race feeling like I've got a firm grip on my running. In the past, I always dreaded the run portion of *triathlons*, but not this time."

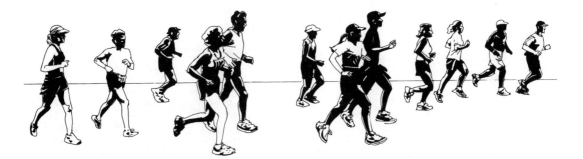

"All runners are not created equal. We do not start with the same genes or have the same time or resources for training. For better or worse, we are all unique. Put things in perspective: Have you ever noticed that faster runners rarely seem satisfied with their performances, while many slower runners wear a perpetual grin on their faces?"

–John "The Penguin" Bingham
Runners' World

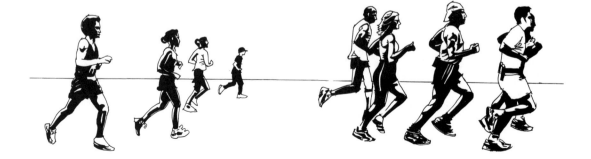

6 THE PROGRAMS

This is the heart of the book. You will be following one of these programs for about six months in preparing for your marathon. If you're a beginner, look at the program on p. 36. If you're with a group, you'll get help in determining which of these time goals is right for you.

Beginner Program

Week #	Mon	Tue	Wed	Thu	Fri	Sat	Sun
1.	walk 30 min	run/walk 30 min	walk 30 min	run/walk 30 min	walk 30 min	off	3 mi run/walk
2.	walk 30 min	run/walk 30 min	walk 30 min	run/walk 30 min	walk 30 min	off	4.5 mi run/walk
3.	walk 30 min	run/walk 30 min	walk 30 min	run/walk 30 min	walk 30 min	off	3 mi run/walk
4.	walk 30 min	run/walk 30 min	walk 30 min	run/walk 30 min	walk 30 min	off	6 mi run/walk
5.	walk 30 min	run/walk 30 min	walk 30 min	run/walk 30 min	walk 30 min	off	7.5 mi run/walk
6.	walk 30 min	run/walk 30 min	walk 30 min	run/walk 30 min	walk 30 min	off	3 mi
7.	walk 30 min	run/walk 30 min	walk 30 min	run/walk 30 min	walk 30 min	off	9 mi
8.	walk 30 min	run/walk 30 min	walk 30 min	run/walk 30 min	walk 30 min	off	3 mi
9.	walk 30 min	run/walk 30 min	walk 30 min	run/walk 30 min	walk 30 min	off	11 mi
10.	walk 30 min	run/walk 30 min	walk 30 min	run/walk 30 min	walk 30 min	off	4 mi
11.	walk 30 min	run/walk 30 min	walk 30 min	run/walk 30 min	walk 30 min	off	13 mi
12.	walk 30 min	run/walk 30 min	walk 30 min	run/walk 30 min	walk 30 min	off	4 mi
13.	walk 30 min	run/walk 30 min	walk 30 min	run/walk 30 min	walk 30 min	off	15 mi
14.	walk 30 min	run/walk 30 min	walk 30 min	run/walk 30 min	walk 30 min	off	4 mi w/MM
15.	walk 30 min	run/walk 30 min	walk 30 min	run/walk 30 min	walk 30 min	off	17 mi
16.	walk 30 min	run/walk 30 min	walk 30 min	run/walk 30 min	walk 30 min	off	4 mi w/MM
17.	walk 30 min	run/walk 30 min	walk 30 min	run/walk 30 min	walk 30 min	off	20 mi
18.	walk 30 min	run/walk 30 min	walk 30 min	run/walk 30 min	walk 30 min	off	6 mi w/MM
19.	walk 30 min	run/walk 30 min	walk 30 min	run/walk 30 min	walk 30 min	off	6 mi
20.	walk 30 min	run/walk 30 min	walk 30 min	run/walk 30 min	walk 30 min	off	23 mi
21.	walk 30 min	run/walk 30 min	walk 30 min	run/walk 30 min	walk 30 min	off	6 mi w/MM
22.	walk 30 min	run/walk 30 min	walk 30 min	run/walk 30 min	walk 30 min	off	6 mi w/MM
23.	walk 30 min	run/walk 30 min	walk 30 min	run/walk 30 min	walk 30 min	off	24–26 mi
24.	walk 30 min	run/walk 30 min	walk 30 min	run/walk 30 min	walk 30 min	off	6 mi
25.	walk 30 min	run/walk 30 min	walk 30 min	run/walk 30 min	walk 30 min	off	6 mi
26.	walk 30 min	off	walk 30 min	off	walk 30 min	off	**The Marathon**
27.	walk 45 min	run/walk 45 min	walk 30–60 min	run/walk 40 min	walk 30–60 min	off	4 mi run/walk
28.	walk 45 min	run/walk 45 min	walk 30–60 min	run/walk 45 min	walk 30–60 min	off	6 mi run/walk
29.	walk 45 min	run/walk 45 min	walk 30–60 min	run/walk 45 min	walk 30–60 min	off	12–20 mi run/walk

Note: This program is for someone who is beginning to run for the first time. It is the bare minimum to get you through a marathon.

- Run slowly enough so that you can carry on a conversation. It's okay to take deep breaths between sentences, but you don't want to "huff and puff" between every word.

- For the first few weeks, you will be doing more walking than running. On every "run/walk" day, walk for 1 minute and jog 15–60 seconds. Every 3–4 weeks you may evaluate how you're feeling. If you want to increase the running, use the "magic mile" to guide you.

- Be sure to do the running portion slow enough at the beginning of every run (especially the long run) so that you'll feel strong at the end. Being conservative here will allow you to recover faster.

- Don't wait to take walk breaks! By alternating walking and running from the beginning, you speed recovery without losing any of the endurance effect of the long run.

- Best results will be achieved when you increase the long run to 26 miles. If your last one is less than this, you must run slowly and take a few more walk breaks during the first 5–10 miles of the marathon itself.

- As the runs get longer, be sure to keep your blood sugar boosted by consuming some blood sugar booster fuel during the long runs. Drink water continuously before and during exercise and with all food. Don't drink more than 20 oz. an hour during long runs.

- The "magic mile" time trial is included as part of the mileage on certain weekends. On the first one, just time yourself. On each successive "MM," try to improve your time, but don't sprint. See p. 108 for more information.

- Above all, HAVE FUN!

"To Finish" Program

Week #	Mon	Tue	Wed	Thu	Fri	Sat	Sun
1.	walk/XT 40 min	run 30–45 min	walk or XT	run 30–45 min	walk or XT	off	3 mi easy
2.	walk/XT 40 min	run 30–45 min	walk or XT	run 30–45 min	walk or XT	off	4.5 mi
3.	walk/XT 40 min	run 30–45 min	walk or XT	run 30–45 min	walk or XT	off	6 mi
4.	walk/XT 40 min	run 30–45 min	walk or XT	run 30–45 min	walk or XT	off	3 mi
5.	walk/XT 40 min	run 30–45 min	walk or XT	run 30–45 min	walk or XT	off	7.5 mi
6.	walk/XT 40 min	run 30–45 min	walk or XT	run 30–45 min	walk or XT	off	4 mi
7.	walk/XT 40 min	run 30–45 min	walk or XT	run 30–45 min	walk or XT	off	9 mi
8.	walk/XT 40 min	run 30–45 min	walk or XT	run 30–45 min	walk or XT	off	4 mi
9.	walk/XT 40 min	run 30–45 min	walk or XT	run 30–45 min	walk or XT	off	11 mi
10.	walk/XT 40 min	run 30–45 min	walk or XT	run 30–45 min	walk or XT	off	5 mi
11.	walk/XT 40 min	run 30–45 min	walk or XT	run 30–45 min	walk or XT	off	13 mi
12.	walk/XT 40 min	run 30–45 min	walk or XT	run 30–45 min	walk or XT	off	5 mi
13.	walk/XT 40 min	run 30–45 min	walk or XT	run 30–45 min	walk or XT	off	15 mi
14.	walk/XT 40 min	run 30–45 min	walk or XT	run 30–45 min	walk or XT	off	6 mi w/MM
15.	walk/XT 40 min	run 30–45 min	walk or XT	run 30–45 min	walk or XT	off	17 mi
16.	walk/XT 40 min	run 30–45 min	walk or XT	run 30–45 min	walk or XT	off	6 mi w/MM
17.	walk/XT 40 min	run 30–45 min	walk or XT	run 30–45 min	walk or XT	off	20 mi
18.	walk/XT 40 min	run 30–45 min	walk or XT	run 30–45 min	walk or XT	off	6 mi w/MM
19.	walk/XT 40 min	run 30–45 min	walk or XT	run 30–45 min	walk or XT	off	7 mi
20.	walk/XT 40 min	run 30–45 min	walk or XT	run 30–45 min	walk or XT	off	23 mi
21.	walk/XT 40 min	run 30–45 min	walk or XT	run 30–45 min	walk or XT	off	6 mi w/MM
22.	walk/XT 40 min	run 30–45 min	walk or XT	run 30–45 min	walk or XT	off	7 mi
23.	walk/XT 40 min	run 30–45 min	walk or XT	run 30–45 min	walk or XT	off	26 mi
24.	walk/XT 40 min	run 30–45 min	walk or XT	run 30–45 min	walk or XT	off	6 mi w/MM
25.	walk/XT 40 min	run 30–45 min	walk or XT	run 30–45 min	walk or XT	off	7 mi
26.	run 40 min	off	run 30 min	off	run/walk 30 min	off	**The Marathon**
27.	walk 45 min	run/walk 30 min	walk 30–60 min	run/walk 45 min	walk 30–60 min	off	4 mi run/walk
28.	walk 45 min	run/walk 45 min	walk 30–60 min	run/walk 45 min	walk 30–60 min	off	6 mi run/walk
29.	walk 45 min	run/walk 45 min	walk 30–60 min	run/walk 45 min	walk 30–60 min	off	12–20 mi run/walk

Note: This program is for someone who has run before and just wants to finish a marathon.

- Every other day you can cross-train (XT) or walk. It's your choice: cross-country ski machines, water running, cycling and any other mode which you find fun and interesting (but non-pounding). You don't have to do the cross training to finish the marathon, but these activities will improve overall fitness.

- Run slowly enough so that you can carry on a conversation. It's okay to take deep breaths between sentences, but you don't want to "huff and puff" between every word. See the "magic mile" section on p. 108 to set a conservative pace and race goal and a run-walk-run strategy.

- Be sure to do the running portion slow enough at the beginning of every run (especially the long run) so that you are strong at the end. Being conservative here will allow you to recover faster.

- When in doubt, slow down the pace and take more walk breaks from the beginning.

- Don't wait to take walk breaks! By alternating walking and running from the beginning, you speed recovery without losing any of the endurance effect of the long run.

- As the runs get longer, be sure to keep your blood sugar boosted by eating a product that works for you. Gradually introduce your system to the nutrients on your long runs (to see if they are easily digestible) and follow the feeding schedule that works for you during the marathon. See "Boosting Blood Sugar" on pp. 147–150.

- Best results will be achieved when you increase the long run to 26 miles. If your last one is less than this, you must run slowly and take a few more walk breaks during the first 5–10 miles of the marathon itself.

Fat-Burning Training

Week #	Mon	Tue	Wed	Thu	Fri	Sat	Sun
1.	30 min walk/jog	XT	30 min walk	XT	30 min walk/jog	walk	3 mi easy
2.	30 min walk/jog	XT	35 min walk/jog	XT	35 min walk/jog	walk	4.5 mi
3.	30 min walk/jog	XT	40 min walk/jog	XT	40 min walk/jog	walk	6 mi
4.	30 min walk/jog	XT	45 min walk/jog	XT	45 min walk/jog	walk	3 mi
5.	30 min walk/jog	XT	45–50 min walk/jog	XT	45–50 min walk/jog	walk	7.5 mi
6.	30 min walk/jog	XT	45–50 min walk/jog	XT	45–50 min walk/jog	walk	4 mi
7.	30 min walk/jog	XT	50–55 min walk/jog	XT	50–55 min walk/jog	walk	9 mi
8.	30 min walk/jog	XT	50–55 min walk/jog	XT	50–55 min walk/jog	walk	4 mi
9.	30 min walk/jog	XT	55–60 min walk/jog	XT	55–60 min walk/jog	walk	11 mi
10.	30 min walk/jog	XT	55–60 min walk/jog	XT	55–60 min walk/jog	walk	4 mi
11.	30 min walk/jog	XT	60–65 min walk/jog	XT	60–65 min walk/jog	walk	13 mi
12.	30 min walk/jog	XT	60–65 min walk/jog	XT	60–65 min walk/jog	walk	4 mi
13.	30 min walk/jog	XT	60–70 min walk/jog	XT	60–70 min walk/jog	walk	15 mi
14.	30 min walk/jog	XT	60–70 min walk/jog	XT	60–70 min walk/jog	walk	4 mi
15.	30 min walk/jog	XT	60–75 min walk/jog	XT	60–75 min walk/jog	walk	17 mi
16.	30 min walk/jog	XT	60–75 min walk/jog	XT	60–75 min walk/jog	walk	4 mi w/MM
17.	30 min walk/jog	XT	60–80 min walk/jog	XT	60–80 min walk/jog	walk	20 mi
18.	30 min walk/jog	XT	60–80 min walk/jog	XT	60–80 min walk/jog	walk	5 mi w/MM
19.	30 min walk/jog	XT	60–85 min walk/jog	XT	60–85 min walk/jog	walk	6 mi
20.	30 min walk/jog	XT	60–85 min walk/jog	XT	60–85 min walk/jog	walk	23 mi
21.	30 min walk/jog	XT	60–90 min walk/jog	XT	60–90 min walk/jog	walk	6 mi w/MM
22.	30 min walk/jog	XT	60–90 min walk/jog	XT	60–90 min walk/jog	walk	6 mi
23.	30 min walk/jog	XT	45–60 min walk/jog	XT	45–60 min walk/jog	walk	26 mi
24.	30 min walk/jog	XT	45–60 min walk/jog	XT	45–60 min walk/jog	walk	6 mi w/MM
25.	30 min walk/jog	XT	45–60 min walk/jog	XT	45–60 min walk/jog	walk	7 mi
26.	30 min walk/jog	XT	45–60 min walk/jog	XT	45–60 min walk/jog	walk	**The Marathon**
27.	30 min walk/jog	XT	45 min walk/jog	XT	45 min walk/jog	walk	4 mi run/walk
28.	30 min walk/jog	XT	60 min walk/jog	XT	60 min walk/jog	walk	6 mi run/walk
29.	30 min walk/jog	XT	60 min walk/jog	XT	60 min walk/jog	walk	12–20 mi run/walk

Note: This program is for someone who is running a marathon as a means of losing weight (fat). *(See pp. 132–139, "Fat Burning as a Way of Life.")*

- Every other day you can cross train or walk; it's your choice. Use cross-country ski machines, cycling, and any other mode that you find fun, interesting, but not pounding. You don't have to do the cross training to finish the marathon, but these activities will improve your overall fitness and burn more fat. It's better to do exercises that build body heat up to a level that you can stand for at least 45 minutes. If this means taking it very easy in the beginning, do so. It's also fine to alternate segments of 10–15 minutes of different exercises but move quickly between segments.

- Be sure that you can carry on a conversation during all of your exercise sessions. This means that you should be exerting yourself at a low enough level that allows you to talk. It's okay to take deep breaths between sentences, but you don't want to "huff and puff" between every word. This is the test for staying aerobic and therefore inside the fat-burning zone.

- Beginners with no exercise background may need to take sit-down breaks of 1–2 minutes for every 4–10 minutes of walking, running and walking, or cross training. If these breaks allow you to do more exercise and recover faster, take them.

- Be sure to do the running portion slowly enough at the beginning of every run (especially the long run) so that you'll be able to continue past the 45-minute mark inside the fat-burning zone (the no-puffing zone). Being conservative here will also speed recovery.

- When in doubt, slow down the pace and take more walk breaks from the beginning. It is the distance covered, not the speed, that determines how much fat you've burned. Slow down, burn more, and feel better during your exercise tomorrow as well as today. Read the "magic mile" section on p. 108, and slow down accordingly.

- Don't wait to take walk breaks! By alternating walking and running from the beginning, you speed recovery without losing any of the endurance benefits of the long run. See "The Galloway Run-Walk-Run Method" on pp. 14–22.

- As the runs get longer, be sure to keep your blood sugar boosted by eating a product that works for you. Gradually introduce your system to the nutrients on your long runs (to see if they are easily digestible) and follow the feeding schedule that works for you during the marathon. See "Boosting Blood Sugar" on pp. 147–150.

- When in doubt, slow down and walk more!

Time-Goal Marathon 4:40

Week #	Mon	Tue	Wed	Thu	Fri	Sat	Sun
1.	XT	40–50 min	20–30 min	XT	40–50 min	off	4–6 hills (5–7 mi)
2.	XT	40–50 min	20–30 min	XT	40–50 min	off	6–7 mi
3.	XT	40–50 min	20–30 min	XT	40–50 min	off	7–8 hills (7.5 mi)
4.	XT	40–50 min	20–30 min	XT	40–50 min	off	9–10 hills (9 mi)
5.	XT	45–50 min	25–35 min	XT	45–50 min	off	4 mi
6.	XT	45–50 min	25–35 min	XT	45–50 min	off	11 mi
7.	XT	45–50 min	25–35 min	XT	45–50 min	off	5 mi
8.	XT	45–50 min	25–35 min	XT	45–50 min	off	13 mi
9.	XT	45–50 min	25–35 min	XT	45–50 min	off	5 mi
10.	XT	45–55 min	25–40 min	XT	45–55 min	off	15 mi easy
11.	XT	45–55 min	25–40 min	XT	45–55 min	off	5 mi w/MM
12.	XT	45–55 min	25–40 min	XT	45–55 min	off	17 mi easy
13.	XT	45–55 min	25–40 min	XT	45–55 min	off	4 × 1 mi
14.	XT	45–55 min	25–40 min	XT	45–55 min	off	20 mi easy
15.	XT	45–55 min	25–40 min	XT	45–55 min	off	6 × 1 mi
16.	XT	45–55 min	25–40 min	XT	45–55 min	off	6 mi w/MM
17.	XT	45–55 min	25–40 min	XT	45–55 min	off	23 mi easy
18.	XT	45–55 min	25–40 min	XT	45–55 min	off	8 × 1 mi
19.	XT	45–55 min	25–40 min	XT	45–55 min	off	6 mi w/MM
20.	XT	45–55 min	25–40 min	XT	45–55 min	off	26 mi easy
21.	XT	45–55 min	25–40 min	XT	45–55 min	off	10 × 1 mi
22.	XT	45–55 min	25–40 min	XT	45–55 min	off	6 mi w/MM
23.	XT	45–55 min	25–40 min	XT	45–55 min	off	28 mi easy
24.	XT	45–55 min	25–40 min	XT	45–55 min	off	12 × 1 mi
25.	XT	40–45 min	20–25 min	XT	40–45 min	off	7 mi
26.	run 40 min	off	run 30 min	off	run 30 min	off	**The Marathon**
27.	walk 45 min	run/walk 30 min	walk 30–60 min	run/walk 40 min	walk 30–60 min	off	7–10 mi run/walk
28.	walk 45 min	run/walk 45 min	walk 30–60 min	run/walk 45 min	walk 30–60 min	off	9–15 mi run/walk
29.	walk 45 min	run/walk 45 min	walk 30–60 min	run/walk 45 min	walk 30–60 min	off	12–20 mi run/walk

- After hill and speed sessions and 5K races you'll see the total mileage recommendation for the day in parentheses. This can be accumulated by adding up the warm-up, the warm-down, hill distance, and any other running during the session.

- On the XT (cross-training) days you can swim, run in the water, use exercise machines such as rowing, cross-country ski, and cycle. Don't use the stair machines. If you miss one of these XT days, don't worry.

- Run the long runs at least 2 minutes per mile slower than you could run a marathon on that day (adjust for heat, humidity, hills, etc.). Follow the instructions in the "magic mile" section. *(See p. 108.)* Slow down by 30 seconds per mile for every 5-degree temperature increase above 60°F.

- Take a 1-minute walk break every 3–5 minutes from the beginning of every long run. On the first few long runs, you may run 5 minutes between breaks. Use the "magic mile" to set pace. Then use the Run-Walk-Run Strategy table *(see p. 20)* to find the right strategy for you for each long run.

- Early in the schedule, hill play is recommended on weekends. Do not sprint. After a relaxed warm-up, do 4–8 accelerations. Then run each hill at about 10K race pace. Keep feet low to the ground and avoid tension in the leg muscles (especially the hamstring). Run up and over the top of the hill, and walk down. Walk more before the next hill if you need more recovery.

- Follow the same warm-up procedure for mile repeats. For a time goal of 4:40, run each mile repeat in 10:15, using a run-walk-run strategy of run 2:30/walk 30 seconds. This prepares you for the pace you'll be running between walk breaks in the marathon. If you're unrealistically optimistic in predicting your marathon goal pace, you'll run the mile repeats too fast and risk over-training and injury. So if this pace causes you to breathe heavily, shift to a slower pace and adjust your marathon goal accordingly. Be sure to walk (don't jog) between mile repeats for 5 minutes.

- Marathon pace running can be done on two other days during the week (Wednesday and Friday). After a slow warm-up, followed by 4–8 acceleration gliders, run 1–3 miles at 10:50, using a run-walk-run ratio of run 2:30/walk 1 minutes. This tells you what it's like to run at marathon goal pace. Make sure that you've recovered from the weekend run, and break up the paced miles with slow jogging between.

- The pace of the Tuesday run should be at least 1 minute per mile slower than marathon goal pace and slower if you're still tired from the weekend session. You may also do a few acceleration gliders on this day, but be careful. Never hesitate to slow down on the Tuesday, Wednesday and Friday runs.

- You have some flexibility on the number of minutes to be run during the week. Never increase the amount more than 10 percent above what you have been doing the week before. Don't hesitate to cut back on some of these days if you're feeling tired from the (hopefully) playful but tiring weekend.

Time-Goal Marathon 4:20

Week #	Mon	Tue	Wed	Thu	Fri	Sat	Sun
1.	XT	40–50 min	20–30 min	XT	40–50 min	off	4–6 hills (5–7 mi)
2.	XT	40–50 min	20–30 min	XT	40–50 min	off	6–7 mi
3.	XT	40–50 min	20–30 min	XT	40–50 min	off	7–8 hills (7.5 mi)
4.	XT	40–50 min	20–30 min	XT	40–50 min	off	9–10 hills (9 mi)
5.	XT	45–50 min	25–35 min	XT	45–50 min	off	4 mi
6.	XT	45–50 min	25–35 min	XT	45–50 min	off	11 mi
7.	XT	45–50 min	25–35 min	XT	45–50 min	off	5 mi
8.	XT	45–50 min	25–35 min	XT	45–50 min	off	13 mi
9.	XT	45–50 min	25–35 min	XT	45–50 min	off	5 mi
10.	XT	45–55 min	25–40 min	XT	45–55 min	off	15 mi easy
11.	XT	45–55 min	25–40 min	XT	45–55 min	off	5 mi w/MM
12.	XT	45–55 min	25–40 min	XT	45–55 min	off	17 mi easy
13.	XT	45–55 min	25–40 min	XT	45–55 min	off	4 x 1 mi
14.	XT	45–55 min	25–40 min	XT	45–55 min	off	20 mi easy
15.	XT	45–55 min	25–40 min	XT	45–55 min	off	6 x 1 mi
16.	XT	45–55 min	25–40 min	XT	45–55 min	off	6 mi w/MM
17.	XT	45–55 min	25–40 min	XT	45–55 min	off	23 mi easy
18.	XT	45–55 min	25–40 min	XT	45–55 min	off	8 x 1 mi
19.	XT	45–55 min	25–40 min	XT	45–55 min	off	6 mi w/MM
20.	XT	45–55 min	25–40 min	XT	45–55 min	off	26 mi easy
21.	XT	45–55 min	25–40 min	XT	45–55 min	off	10 x 1 mi
22.	XT	45–55 min	25–40 min	XT	45–55 min	off	6 mi w/MM
23.	XT	45–55 min	25–40 min	XT	45–55 min	off	28 mi easy
24.	XT	45–55 min	25–40 min	XT	45–55 min	off	12 x 1 mi
25.	XT	40–45 min	20–25 min	XT	40–45 min	off	7 mi
26.	run 40 min	off	run 30 min	off	run 30 min	off	**The Marathon**
27.	walk 45 min	run/walk 30 min	walk 30–60 min	run/walk 45 min	walk 30–60 min	off	4 mi run/walk
28.	walk 45 min	run/walk 45 min	walk 30–60 min	run/walk 45 min	walk 30–60 min	off	6 mi run/walk
29.	walk 45 min	run/walk 45 min	walk 30–60 min	run/walk 45 min	walk 30–60 min	off	12–20 mi run/walk

- After hill and speed sessions and 5K races you'll see the total mileage recommendation for the day in parentheses. This can be accumulated by adding up the warm-up, the warm-down, hill distance, and any other running during the session.
- On the XT (cross-training) days you can swim, run in the water, use exercise machines such as rowing, cross-country ski, and cycle. Don't use the stair machines. If you miss one of these XT days, don't worry.

- Run the long runs at least 2 minutes per mile slower than you could run a marathon on that day (adjust for heat, humidity, hills, etc.). Follow the instructions in the "magic mile" section. *(See p. 108.)* Slow down by 30 seconds per mile for every 5-degree temperature increase above 60°F.

- Take a 1-minute walk break every 3–5 minutes from the beginning of every long run. On the first few long runs, you may run 5 minutes between breaks. Use the "magic mile" to set pace. Then use the Run-Walk-Run Strategy table *(see p. 20)* to find the right strategy for you for each long run.

- Early in the schedule, hill play is recommended on weekends. Do not sprint. After a relaxed warm-up, do 4–8 accelerations. Then run each hill at about 10K race pace. Keep feet low to the ground and avoid tension in the leg muscles (especially the hamstring). Run up and over the top of the hill, and walk down. Walk more before the next hill if you need more recovery.

- Follow the same warm-up procedure for mile repeats. For a time goal of 4:20, run each mile repeat in 9:30, using a run-walk-run strategy of run 3 minutes/walk 30 seconds. This prepares you for the pace you'll be running between walk breaks in the marathon. If you're unrealistically optimistic in predicting your marathon goal pace, you'll run the mile repeats too fast and risk over-training and injury. So if this pace causes you to breathe heavily, shift to a slower pace and adjust your marathon goal accordingly. Be sure to walk (don't jog) between mile repeats for 5 minutes.

- Marathon pace running can be done on two other days during the week (Wednesday and Friday). After a slow warm-up, followed by 4–8 acceleration gliders, run 1–3 miles at 10 minutes per mile, using a run-walk-run strategy of 3/1. This tells you what it's like to run at marathon goal pace. Make sure that you've recovered from the weekend run, and break up the paced miles with slow jogging between.

- The pace of the Tuesday run should be at least 1 minute per mile slower than marathon goal pace and slower if you're still tired from the weekend session. You may also do a few acceleration gliders on this day, but be careful. Never hesitate to slow down on the Tuesday, Wednesday and Friday runs.

- You have some flexibility on the number of minutes to be run during the week. Never increase the amount more than 10 percent above what you have been doing the week before. Don't hesitate to cut back on some of these days if you're feeling tired from the (hopefully) playful but tiring weekend.

Time-Goal Marathon 4:00

Week #	Mon	Tue	Wed	Thu	Fri	Sat	Sun
1.	XT	40–50 min	20–30 min	XT	40–50 min	off	4–6 hills (5–7 mi)
2.	XT	40–50 min	20–30 min	XT	40–50 min	off	6–7 mi
3.	XT	40–50 min	20–30 min	XT	40–50 min	off	7–8 hills (7.5 mi)
4.	XT	40–50 min	20–30 min	XT	40–50 min	off	9–10 hills (9 mi)
5.	XT	45–50 min	25–35 min	XT	45–50 min	off	4 mi
6.	XT	45–50 min	25–35 min	XT	45–50 min	off	11 mi
7.	XT	45–50 min	25–35 min	XT	45–50 min	off	5 mi
8.	XT	45–50 min	25–35 min	XT	45–50 min	off	13 mi
9.	XT	45–50 min	25–35 min	XT	45–50 min	off	5 mi
10.	XT	45–55 min	25–40 min	XT	45–55 min	off	15 mi easy
11.	XT	45–55 min	25–40 min	XT	45–55 min	off	5 mi w/MM
12.	XT	45–55 min	25–40 min	XT	45–55 min	off	17 mi easy
13.	XT	45–55 min	25–40 min	XT	45–55 min	off	4 x 1 mi
14.	XT	45–55 min	25–40 min	XT	45–55 min	off	20 mi easy
15.	XT	45–55 min	25–40 min	XT	45–55 min	off	6 x 1 mi
16.	XT	45–55 min	25–40 min	XT	45–55 min	off	6 mi w/MM
17.	XT	45–55 min	25–40 min	XT	45–55 min	off	23 mi easy
18.	XT	45–55 min	25–40 min	XT	45–55 min	off	8 x 1 mi
19.	XT	45–55 min	25–40 min	XT	45–55 min	off	6 mi w/MM
20.	XT	45–55 min	25–40 min	XT	45–55 min	off	26 mi easy
21.	XT	45–55 min	25–40 min	XT	45–55 min	off	10 x 1 mi
22.	XT	45–55 min	25–40 min	XT	45–55 min	off	6 mi w/MM
23.	XT	45–55 min	25–40 min	XT	45–55 min	off	28 mi easy
24.	XT	45–55 min	25–40 min	XT	45–55 min	off	12 x 1 mi
25.	XT	40–45 min	20–25 min	XT	40–45 min	off	7 mi
26.	run 40 min	off	run 30 min	off	run 30 min	off	**The Marathon**
27.	walk 45 min	run/walk 30 min	walk 30–60 min	run/walk 45 min	walk 30–60 min	off	4 mi run/walk
28.	walk 45 min	run/walk 45 min	walk 30–60 min	run/walk 45 min	walk 30–60 min	off	6 mi run/walk
29.	walk 45 min	run/walk 45 min	walk 30–60 min	run/walk 45 min	walk 30–60 min	off	12–20 mi run/walk

- After hill and speed sessions and 5K races you'll see the total mileage recommendation for the day in parentheses. This can be accumulated by adding up the warm-up, the warm-down, hill distance, and any other running during the session.

- On the XT (cross-training) days you can swim, run in the water, use exercise machines such as rowing, cross-country ski, and cycle. Don't use the stair machines. If you miss one of these XT days, don't worry.

- Run the long runs at least 2 minutes per mile slower than you could run a marathon on that day (adjust for heat, humidity, hills, etc.). Follow the instructions in the "magic mile" section. *(See p. 108.)* Slow down by 30 seconds per mile for every 5-degree temperature increase above 60°F.

- Take a 1-minute walk break every 3–5 minutes from the beginning of every long run. On the first few long runs, you may run 5 minutes between breaks. Use the "magic mile" to set pace. Then use the Run-Walk-Run Strategy table *(see p. 20)* to find the right strategy for you for each long run.

- Early in the schedule, hill play is recommended on weekends. Do not sprint. After a relaxed warm-up, do 4–8 accelerations. Then run each hill at about 10K race pace. Keep feet low to the ground and avoid tension in the leg muscles (especially the hamstring). Run up and over the top of the hill, and walk down. Walk more before the next hill if you need more recovery.

- Follow the same warm-up procedure for mile repeats. For a time goal of 4:00, run each mile repeat in 8:40, using a run-walk-run strategy of run 4 minutes/walk 30 seconds. This prepares you for the pace you'll be running between walk breaks in the marathon. If you're unrealistically optimistic in predicting your marathon goal pace, you'll run the mile repeats too fast and risk over-training and injury. So if this pace causes you to breathe heavily, shift to a slower pace and adjust your marathon goal accordingly. Be sure to walk (don't jog) between mile repeats for at least 4 minutes.

- Marathon pace running can be done on two other days during the week (Wednesday and Friday). After a slow warm-up, followed by 4–8 acceleration gliders, run 1–3 miles at 9 minutes per mile, using a run-walk-run strategy of run 4 minutes/walk 1 minute. This tells you what it's like to run at marathon goal pace. Make sure that you've recovered from the weekend run, and break up the paced miles with slow jogging between.

- The pace of the Tuesday run should be at least 1 minute per mile slower than marathon goal pace and slower if you're still tired from the weekend session. You may also do a few acceleration gliders on this day, but be careful. Never hesitate to slow down on the Tuesday, Wednesday and Friday runs.

- You have some flexibility on the number of minutes to be run during the week. Never increase the amount more than 10 percent above what you have been doing the week before. Don't hesitate to cut back on some of these days if you're feeling tired from the (hopefully) playful but tiring weekend.

Time-Goal Marathon 3:45

Week #	Mon	Tue	Wed	Thu	Fri	Sat	Sun
1.	XT	40–50 min	20–30 min	XT	40–50 min	off	4–6 hills (5–7 mi)
2.	XT	40–50 min	20–30 min	XT	40–50 min	off	6–7 mi
3.	XT	40–50 min	20–30 min	XT	40–50 min	off	7–8 hills (7.5 mi)
4.	XT	40–50 min	20–30 min	XT	40–50 min	off	9–10 hills (9 mi)
5.	XT	45–50 min	25–35 min	XT	45–50 min	off	6 mi
6.	XT	45–50 min	25–35 min	XT	45–50 min	off	11 mi
7.	XT	45–50 min	25–35 min	XT	45–50 min	off	6 mi
8.	XT	45–50 min	25–35 min	XT	45–50 min	off	13 mi
9.	XT	45–50 min	25–35 min	XT	45–50 min	off	6 mi
10.	XT	45–55 min	25–40 min	XT	45–55 min	off	15 mi easy
11.	XT	45–55 min	25–40 min	XT	45–55 min	off	4 × 1 mi
12.	XT	45–55 min	25–40 min	XT	45–55 min	off	17 mi easy
13.	XT	45–55 min	25–40 min	XT	45–55 min	off	6 × 1 mi
14.	XT	45–55 min	25–50 min	XT	45–65 min	off	20 mi easy
15.	XT	45–55 min	25–50 min	XT	45–65 min	off	8 × 1 mi
16.	XT	45–55 min	25–50 min	XT	45–65 min	off	7 mi w/MM
17.	XT	45–55 min	25–50 min	XT	45–65 min	off	23 mi easy
18.	XT	45–55 min	25–50 min	XT	45–65 min	off	10 × 1 mi
19.	XT	45–55 min	25–60 min	XT	45–75 min	off	7 mi w/MM
20.	XT	45–55 min	25–60 min	XT	45–75 min	off	26 mi easy
21.	XT	45–55 min	25–60 min	XT	45–75 min	off	12 × 1 mi
22.	XT	45–55 min	25–60 min	XT	45–75 min	off	7 mi w/MM
23.	XT	45–55 min	25–60 min	XT	45–75 min	off	29 mi easy
24.	XT	45–55 min	25–60 min	XT	45–75 min	off	14 × 1 mi
25.	XT	40–45 min	20–25 min	XT	40–45 min	off	7 mi
26.	run 40 min	off	run 30 min	off	run 30 min	off	**The Marathon**
27.	walk 45 min	run/walk 30 min	walk 30–60 min	run/walk 40 min	walk 30–60 min	off	4 mi run/walk
28.	walk 45 min	run/walk 45 min	walk 30–60 min	run/walk 45 min	walk 30–60 min	off	6 mi run/walk
29.	walk 45 min	run/walk 45 min	walk 30–60 min	run/walk 45 min	walk 30–60 min	off	12–20 mi run/walk

- After hill and speed sessions and 5K races you'll see the total mileage recommendation for the day in parentheses. This can be accumulated by adding up the warm-up, the warm-down, hill distance, and any other running during the session.

- On the XT (cross-training) days you can swim, run in the water, use exercise machines such as rowing, cross-country ski, and cycle. Don't use the stair machines. If you miss one of these XT days, don't worry.

- Run the long runs at least 2 minutes per mile slower than you could run a marathon on that day (adjust for heat, humidity, hills, etc.). Follow the instructions in the "magic mile" section. *(See p. 108.)* Slow down by 30 seconds per mile for every 5-degree temperature increase above 60°F.

- Take a 1-minute walk break every 3–5 minutes from the beginning of every long run. On the first few long runs, you may run 5 minutes between breaks. Use the "magic mile" to set pace. Then use the Run-Walk-Run Strategy table *(see p. 20)* to find the right strategy for you for each long run.

- Early in the schedule, hill play is recommended on weekends. Do not sprint. After a relaxed warm-up, do 4–8 accelerations. Then run each hill at about 10K race pace. Keep feet low to the ground and avoid tension in the leg muscles (especially the hamstring). Run up and over the top of the hill, and walk down. Walk more before the next hill if you need more recovery.

- Follow the same warm-up procedure for mile repeats. For a time goal of 3:45, run each mile repeat in 8:05, using a run-walk-run strategy of run 4 minutes/walk 22 seconds. This prepares you for the pace you'll be running between walk breaks in the marathon. If you're unrealistically optimistic in predicting your marathon goal pace, you'll run the mile repeats too fast and risk over-training and injury. So if this pace causes you to breathe heavily, shift to a slower pace and adjust your marathon goal accordingly. Be sure to walk (don't jog) between mile repeats for at least 4 minutes.

- Marathon pace running can be done on two other days during the week (Wednesday and Friday). After a slow warm-up, followed by 4–8 acceleration gliders, run 3 miles at 8:30 minutes per mile, using a run-walk-run strategy of run 4 minutes/walk 45 seconds. This tells you what it's like to run at marathon goal pace. Make sure that you've recovered from the weekend run, and break up the paced miles with slow jogging between.

- The pace of the Tuesday run should be at least 1 minute per mile slower than marathon goal pace and slower if you're still tired from the weekend session. You may also do a few acceleration gliders on this day, but be careful. Never hesitate to slow down on the Tuesday, Wednesday and Friday runs.

- You have some flexibility on the number of minutes to be run during the week. Never increase the amount more than 10 percent above what you have been doing the week before. Don't hesitate to cut back on some of these days if you're feeling tired from the (hopefully) playful but tiring weekend.

Time-Goal Marathon 3:30

Week #	Mon	Tue	Wed	Thu	Fri	Sat	Sun
1.	XT	40–50 min	20–30 min	XT	40–50 min	off	4–6 hills (5–7 mi)
2.	XT	40–50 min	20–30 min	XT	40–50 min	off	6–7 mi
3.	XT	40–50 min	20–30 min	XT	40–50 min	off	7–8 hills (7.5 mi)
4.	XT	40–50 min	20–30 min	XT	40–50 min	off	9–10 hills (9 mi)
5.	XT	45–50 min	25–35 min	XT	45–50 min	off	6 mi
6.	XT	45–50 min	25–35 min	XT	45–50 min	off	11 mi
7.	XT	45–50 min	25–35 min	XT	45–50 min	off	6 mi
8.	XT	45–50 min	25–35 min	XT	45–50 min	off	13 mi
9.	XT	45–50 min	25–35 min	XT	45–50 min	off	6 mi
10.	XT	45–55 min	25–40 min	XT	45–55 min	off	15 mi easy
11.	XT	45–55 min	25–40 min	XT	45–55 min	off	4 × 1 mi
12.	XT	45–55 min	25–40 min	XT	45–55 min	off	17 mi easy
13.	XT	45–55 min	25–40 min	XT	45–55 min	off	6 × 1 mi
14.	XT	45–55 min	25–50 min	XT	45–65 min	off	20 mi easy
15.	XT	45–55 min	25–50 min	XT	45–65 min	off	8 × 1 mi
16.	XT	45–55 min	25–50 min	XT	45–65 min	off	7 mi w/MM
17.	XT	45–55 min	25–50 min	XT	45–65 min	off	23 mi easy
18.	XT	45–55 min	25–50 min	XT	45–65 min	off	10 × 1 mi
19.	XT	45–55 min	25–60 min	XT	45–75 min	off	7 mi w/MM
20.	XT	45–55 min	25–60 min	XT	45–75 min	off	26 mi easy
21.	XT	45–55 min	25–60 min	XT	45–75 min	off	12 × 1 mi
22.	XT	45–55 min	25–60 min	XT	45–75 min	off	7 mi w/MM
23.	XT	45–55 min	25–60 min	XT	45–75 min	off	29 mi easy
24.	XT	45–55 min	25–60 min	XT	45–75 min	off	14 × 1 mi
25.	XT	40–45 min	20–25 min	XT	40–45 min	off	7 mi
26.	run 40 min	off	run 30 min	off	run 30 min	off	**The Marathon**
27.	walk 45 min	run/walk 30 min	walk 30–60 min	run/walk 40 min	walk 30–60 min	off	4 mi run/walk
28.	walk 45 min	run/walk 45 min	walk 30–60 min	run/walk 45 min	walk 30–60 min	off	6 mi run/walk
29.	walk 45 min	run/walk 45 min	walk 30–60 min	run/walk 45 min	walk 30–60 min	off	12–20 mi run/walk

- After hill and speed sessions and 5K races you'll see the total mileage recommendation for the day in parentheses. This can be accumulated by adding up the warm-up, the warm-down, hill distance, and any other running during the session.
- On the XT (cross-training) days you can swim, run in the water, use exercise machines such as rowing, cross-country ski, and cycle. Don't use the stair machines. If you miss one of these XT days, don't worry.

- Run the long runs at least 2 minutes per mile slower than you could run a marathon on that day (adjust for heat, humidity, hills, etc.). Follow the instructions in the "magic mile" section. *(See p. 108.)* Slow down by 30 seconds per mile for every 5-degree temperature increase above 60°F.

- Take a 1-minute walk break every 3–5 minutes from the beginning of every long run. On the first few long runs, you may run 5 minutes between breaks. Use the "magic mile" to set pace. Then use the Run-Walk-Run Strategy table *(see p. 20)* to find the right strategy for you for each long run.

- Early in the schedule, hill play is recommended on weekends. Do not sprint. After a relaxed warm-up, do 4–8 accelerations. Then run each hill at about 10K race pace. Keep feet low to the ground and avoid tension in the leg muscles (especially the hamstring). Run up and over the top of the hill, and walk down. Walk more before the next hill if you need more recovery.

- Follow the same warm-up procedure for mile repeats. For a time goal of 3:30, run each mile repeat in 7:30, using a run-walk-run strategy of run 4 minutes/walk 15 seconds. This prepares you for the pace you'll be running between walk breaks in the marathon. If you're unrealistically optimistic in predicting your marathon goal pace, you'll run the mile repeats too fast and risk over-training and injury. So if this pace causes you to breathe heavily, shift to a slower pace and adjust your marathon goal accordingly. Be sure to walk (don't jog) between mile repeats for at least 4 minutes.

- Marathon pace running can be done on two other days during the week (Wednesday and Friday). After a slow warm-up, followed by 4–8 acceleration gliders, run 3 miles at 8 minutes per mile, using a run-walk-run strategy of run 4 minutes/walk 30 seconds. This tells you what it's like to run at marathon goal pace. Make sure that you've recovered from the weekend run, and break up the paced miles with slow jogging between.

- The pace of the Tuesday run should be at least 1 minute per mile slower than marathon goal pace and slower if you're still tired from the weekend session. You may also do a few acceleration gliders on this day, but be careful. Never hesitate to slow down on the Tuesday, Wednesday and Friday runs.

- You have some flexibility on the number of minutes to be run during the week. Never increase the amount more than 10 percent above what you have been doing the week before. Don't hesitate to cut back on some of these days if you're feeling tired from the (hopefully) playful but tiring weekend.

Time-Goal Marathon 3:15

Week #	Mon	Tue	Wed	Thu	Fri	Sat	Sun
1.	XT	40–50 min	20–30 min	XT	40–50 min	off	4–6 hills (5–7 mi)
2.	XT	40–50 min	20–30 min	XT	40–50 min	off	6–7 mi
3.	XT	40–50 min	20–30 min	XT	40–50 min	off	7–8 hills (7.5 mi)
4.	XT	40–50 min	20–30 min	XT	40–50 min	off	9–10 hills (9 mi)
5.	XT	45–50 min	25–35 min	XT	45–50 min	off	6 mi
6.	XT	45–50 min	25–35 min	XT	45–50 min	off	11 mi
7.	XT	45–50 min	25–35 min	XT	45–50 min	off	6 mi
8.	XT	45–50 min	25–35 min	XT	45–50 min	off	13 mi
9.	XT	45–50 min	25–35 min	XT	45–50 min	off	6 mi
10.	XT	45–55 min	25–40 min	XT	45–55 min	off	15 mi easy
11.	XT	45–55 min	25–40 min	XT	45–55 min	off	4 × 1 mi
12.	XT	45–55 min	25–40 min	XT	45–55 min	off	17 mi easy
13.	XT	45–55 min	25–40 min	XT	45–55 min	off	6 × 1 mi
14.	XT	45–55 min	25–50 min	XT	45–65 min	off	20 mi easy
15.	XT	45–55 min	25–50 min	XT	45–65 min	off	8 × 1 mi
16.	XT	45–55 min	25–50 min	XT	45–65 min	off	7 mi w/MM
17.	XT	45–55 min	25–50 min	XT	45–65 min	off	23 mi easy
18.	XT	45–55 min	25–50 min	XT	45–65 min	off	10 × 1 mi
19.	XT	45–55 min	25–60 min	XT	45–75 min	off	7 mi w/MM
20.	XT	45–55 min	25–60 min	XT	45–75 min	off	26 mi easy
21.	XT	45–55 min	25–60 min	XT	45–75 min	off	12 × 1 mi
22.	XT	45–55 min	25–60 min	XT	45–75 min	off	7 mi w/MM
23.	XT	45–55 min	25–60 min	XT	45–75 min	off	29 mi easy
24.	XT	45–55 min	25–60 min	XT	45–75 min	off	14 × 1 mi
25.	XT	40–45 min	20–25 min	XT	40–45 min	off	7 mi
26.	run 40 min	off	run 30 min	off	run 30 min	off	**The Marathon**
27.	walk 45 min	run/walk 30 min	walk 30–60 min	run/walk 40 min	walk 30–60 min	off	4 mi run/walk
28.	walk 45 min	run/walk 45 min	walk 30–60 min	run/walk 45 min	walk 30–60 min	off	6 mi run/walk
29.	walk 45 min	run/walk 45 min	walk 30–60 min	run/walk 45 min	walk 30–60 min	off	12–20 mi run/walk

- After hill and speed sessions and 5K races you'll see the total mileage recommendation for the day in parentheses. This can be accumulated by adding up the warm-up, the warm-down, hill distance, and any other running during the session.
- On the XT (cross-training) days you can swim, run in the water, use exercise machines such as rowing, cross-country ski, and cycle. Don't use the stair machines. If you miss one of these XT days, don't worry.

- Run the long runs at least 2 minutes per mile slower than you could run a marathon on that day (adjust for heat, humidity, hills, etc.). Follow the instructions in the "magic mile" section. *(See p. 108.)* Slow down by 30 seconds per mile for every 5-degree temperature increase above 60°F.

- Take a 1-minute walk break every 3–5 minutes from the beginning of every long run. On the first few long runs, you may run 5 minutes between breaks. Use the "magic mile" to set pace. Then use the Run-Walk-Run Strategy table *(see p. 20)* to find the right strategy for you for each long run.

- Early in the schedule, hill play is recommended on weekends. Do not sprint. After a relaxed warm-up, do 4–8 accelerations. Then run each hill at about 10K race pace. Keep feet low to the ground and avoid tension in the leg muscles (especially the hamstring). Run up and over the top of the hill, and walk down. Walk more before the next hill if you need more recovery.

- Follow the same warm-up procedure for mile repeats. For a time goal of 3:15, run each mile repeat in 7:00, using a run-walk-run strategy of run 5 minutes/walk 15 seconds. This prepares you for the pace you'll be running between walk breaks in the marathon. If you're unrealistically optimistic in predicting your marathon goal pace, you'll run the mile repeats too fast and risk over-training and injury. So if this pace causes you to breathe heavily, shift to a slower pace and adjust your marathon goal accordingly. Be sure to walk (don't jog) between mile repeats for at least 4 minutes.

- Marathon pace running can be done on two other days during the week (Wednesday and Friday). After a slow warm-up, followed by 4–8 acceleration gliders, run 3 miles at 7:25 pace, using a run-walk-run strategy of run 5 minutes/walk 30 seconds, or run a mile/walk 45 seconds. This tells you what it's like to run at marathon goal pace. Make sure that you've recovered from the weekend run, and break up the paced miles with slow jogging between.

- The pace of the Tuesday run should be at least 1 minute per mile slower than marathon goal pace and slower if you're still tired from the weekend session. You may also do a few acceleration gliders on this day, but be careful. Never hesitate to slow down on the Tuesday, Wednesday and Friday runs.

- You have some flexibility on the number of minutes to be run during the week. Never increase the amount more than 10 percent above what you have been doing the week before. Don't hesitate to cut back on some of these days if you're feeling tired from the (hopefully) playful but tiring weekend.

Time-Goal Marathon 2:59

Week #	Mon	Tue	Wed	Thu	Fri	Sat	Sun
1.	XT	40–50 min	20–30 min	XT	40–50 min	off	4–6 hills (5–7 mi)
2.	XT	40–50 min	20–30 min	XT	40–50 min	off	6–7 mi
3.	XT	40–50 min	20–30 min	XT	40–50 min	off	7–8 hills (7.5 mi)
4.	XT	40–50 min	20–30 min	XT	40–50 min	off	9–10 hills (9 mi)
5.	XT	45–50 min	25–35 min	XT	45–50 min	off	6 mi
6.	XT	45–50 min	25–35 min	XT	45–50 min	off	11 mi
7.	XT	45–50 min	25–35 min	XT	45–50 min	off	6 mi
8.	XT	45–50 min	25–35 min	XT	45–50 min	off	13 mi
9.	XT	45–50 min	25–35 min	XT	45–50 min	off	6 mi
10.	XT	45–55 min	25–40 min	XT	45–55 min	off	15 mi easy
11.	XT	45–55 min	25–40 min	XT	45–55 min	off	4 × 1 mi
12.	XT	45–55 min	25–40 min	XT	45–55 min	off	17 mi easy
13.	XT	45–55 min	25–40 min	XT	45–55 min	off	6 × 1 mi
14.	XT	45–55 min	25–50 min	XT	45–65 min	off	20 mi easy
15.	XT	45–55 min	25–50 min	XT	45–65 min	off	8 × 1 mi
16.	XT	45–55 min	25–50 min	XT	45–65 min	off	7 mi w/MM
17.	XT	45–55 min	25–50 min	XT	45–65 min	off	23 mi easy
18.	XT	45–55 min	25–50 min	XT	45–65 min	off	10 × 1 mi
19.	XT	45–55 min	25–60 min	XT	45–75 min	off	7 mi w/MM
20.	XT	45–55 min	25–60 min	XT	45–75 min	off	26 mi easy
21.	XT	45–55 min	25–60 min	XT	45–75 min	off	12 × 1 mi
22.	XT	45–55 min	25–60 min	XT	45–75 min	off	7 mi w/MM
23.	XT	45–55 min	25–60 min	XT	45–75 min	off	29 mi easy
24.	XT	45–55 min	25–60 min	XT	45–75 min	off	14 × 1 mi
25.	XT	40–45 min	20–25 min	XT	40–45 min	off	7 mi
26.	run 40 min	off	run 30 min	off	run 30 min	off	**The Marathon**
27.	walk 45 min	run/walk 30 min	walk 30–60 min	run/walk 40 min	walk 30–60 min	off	4 mi run/walk
28.	walk 45 min	run/walk 45 min	walk 30–60 min	run/walk 45 min	walk 30–60 min	off	6 mi run/walk
29.	walk 45 min	run/walk 45 min	walk 30–60 min	run/walk 45 min	walk 30–60 min	off	12–20 mi run/walk

- After hill and speed sessions and 5K races you'll see the total mileage recommendation for the day in parentheses. This can be accumulated by adding up the warm-up, the warm-down, hill distance, and any other running during the session.
- On the XT (cross-training) days you can swim, run in the water, use exercise machines such as rowing, cross-country ski, and cycle. Don't use the stair machines. If you miss one of these XT days, don't worry.

- Run the long runs at least 2 minutes per mile slower than you could run a marathon on that day (adjust for heat, humidity, hills, etc.). Follow the instructions in the "magic mile" section. *(See p. 108.)* Slow down by 30 seconds per mile for every 5-degree temperature increase above 60°F.

- Take a 1-minute walk break every 3–5 minutes from the beginning of every long run. On the first few long runs, you may run 5 minutes between breaks. Use the "magic mile" to set pace. Then use the Run-Walk-Run Strategy table *(see p. 20)* to find the right strategy for you for each long run.

- Early in the schedule, hill play is recommended on weekends. Do not sprint. After a relaxed warm-up, do 4–8 accelerations. Then run each hill at about 10K race pace. Keep feet low to the ground and avoid tension in the leg muscles (especially the hamstring). Run up and over the top of the hill, and walk down. Walk more before the next hill if you need more recovery.

- Follow the same warm-up procedure for mile repeats. For a time goal of 2:59, run each mile repeat in 6:25. This prepares you for the pace you'll be running between walk breaks in the marathon. If you're unrealistically optimistic in predicting your marathon goal pace, you'll run the mile repeats too fast and risk over-training and injury. So if this pace causes you to breathe heavily, shift to a slower pace and adjust your marathon goal accordingly. Be sure to walk (don't jog) between mile repeats for at least 4 minutes.

- Marathon pace running can be done on two other days during the week (Wednesday and Friday). After a slow warm-up, followed by 4–8 acceleration gliders, run 3 miles at 6:50 pace, taking a 20- to 30-second walk break each mile. This tells you what it's like to run at marathon goal pace. Make sure that you've recovered from the weekend run, and break up the paced miles with slow jogging between. Hopefully your legs will feel good enough to do 1-2 of these marathon pace miles on the Wednesday and Friday before your marathon (unless the marathon is on Saturday, in which case shift these days to Tuesday and Thursday.

- The pace of the Tuesday run should be at least 1 minute per mile slower than marathon goal pace and slower if you're still tired from the weekend session. You may also do a few acceleration gliders on this day, but be careful. Never hesitate to slow down on the Tuesday, Wednesday and Friday runs.

- You have some flexibility on the number of minutes to be run during the week. Never increase the amount more than 10 percent above what you have been doing the week before. Don't hesitate to cut back on some of these days if you're feeling tired from the (hopefully) playful but tiring weekend.

Time-Goal Marathon 2:39

Week #	Mon	Tue	Wed	Thu	Fri	Sat	Sun
1.	XT	40–55 min	20–50 min	XT	40–55 min	off	4–6 hills (5–7 mi)
2.	XT	40–60 min	20–50 min	XT	40–60 min	off	6–7 mi
3.	XT	40–65 min	20–50 min	XT	40–60 min	off	7–8 hills (7.5 mi)
4.	XT	40–65 min	20–50 min	XT	40–60 min	off	9–10 hills (9 mi)
5.	XT	45–75 min	25–55 min	XT	45–65 min	off	6 mi
6.	XT	45–80 min	25–55 min	XT	45–65 min	off	12 mi
7.	XT	45–80 min	25–55 min	XT	45–70 min	off	6 mi
8.	XT	45–80 min	25–55 min	XT	45–75 min	off	14 mi
9.	XT	45–80 min	25–55 min	XT	45–80 min	off	6 mi
10.	XT	45–85 min	25–60 min	XT	45–80 min	off	16 mi easy
11.	XT	45–85 min	25–60 min	XT	45–85 min	off	4 × 1 mi
12.	XT	45–85 min	25–60 min	XT	45–85 min	off	18 mi easy
13.	XT	45–85 min	25–60 min	XT	45–85 min	off	6 × 1 mi
14.	XT	45–85 min	25–60 min	XT	45–85 min	off	21 mi easy
15.	XT	45–85 min	25–60 min	XT	45–85 min	off	8 × 1 mi
16.	XT	45–85 min	25–60 min	XT	45–85 min	off	7 mi w/MM
17.	XT	45–85 min	25–60 min	XT	45–85 min	off	24 mi easy
18.	XT	45–85 min	25–60 min	XT	45–85 min	off	10 × 1 mi
19.	XT	45–85 min	25–60 min	XT	45–85 min	off	7 mi w/MM
20.	XT	45–85 min	25–60 min	XT	45–85 min	off	27 mi easy
21.	XT	45–85 min	25–60 min	XT	45–85 min	off	12 × 1 mi
22.	XT	45–85 min	25–60 min	XT	45–85 min	off	7 mi w/MM
23.	XT	45–75 min	25–60 min	XT	45–75 min	off	30 mi easy
24.	XT	45–55 min	25–50 min	XT	45–55 min	off	14 × 1 mi
25.	XT	40 min	20–25 min	XT	40 min	off	7 mi
26.	run 40 min	off	run 30 min	off	run 30 min	off	**The Marathon**
27.	walk 45 min	run/walk 30 min	walk 30–60 min	run/walk 40 min	walk 30–60 min	off	4 mi run/walk
28.	walk 45 min	run/walk 45 min	walk 30–60 min	run/walk 45 min	walk 30–60 min	off	6 mi run/walk
29.	walk 45 min	run/walk 45 min	walk 30–60 min	run/walk 45 min	walk 30–60 min	off	12–20 mi run/walk

- After hill and speed sessions and 5K races you'll see the total mileage recommendation for the day in parentheses. This can be accumulated by adding up the warm-up, the warm-down, hill distance, and any other running during the session.

- On the XT (cross-training) days you can swim, run in the water, use exercise machines such as rowing, cross-country ski, and cycle. Don't use the stair machines. If you miss one of these XT days, don't worry.

- Run the long runs at least 2 minutes per mile slower than you could run a marathon on that day (adjust for heat, humidity, hills, etc.). Follow the instructions in the "magic mile" section. *(See p. 108.)* Slow down by 30 seconds per mile for every 5-degree temperature increase above 60°F.

- Take a 1-minute walk break every 3–5 minutes from the beginning of every long run. On the first few long runs, you may run 5 minutes between breaks. Use the "magic mile" to set pace. Then use the Run-Walk-Run Strategy table *(see p. 20)* to find the right strategy for you for each long run.

- Early in the schedule, hill play is recommended on weekends. Do not sprint. After a relaxed warm-up, do 4–8 accelerations. Then run each hill at about 10K race pace. Keep feet low to the ground and avoid tension in the leg muscles (especially the hamstring). Run up and over the top of the hill, and walk down. Walk more before the next hill if you need more recovery.

- Follow the same warm-up procedure for mile repeats. For a time goal of 2:39, run each mile repeat in 5:30. This prepares you for the pace you'll be running between walk breaks in the marathon. If you're unrealistically optimistic in predicting your marathon goal pace, you'll run the mile repeats too fast and risk over-training and injury. So if this pace causes you to breathe heavily, shift to a slower pace and adjust your marathon goal accordingly. Be sure to walk (don't jog) between mile repeats for at least 4 minutes.

- Marathon pace running can be done on two other days during the week (Wednesday and Friday). After a slow warm-up, followed by 4–8 acceleration gliders, run 2–5 miles at 5:50 pace, taking a 20-second walk break each mile. This tells you what it's like to run at marathon goal pace. Make sure that you've recovered from the weekend run, and break up the paced miles with slow jogging between. Hopefully your legs will feel good enough to do 1–2 of these marathon pace miles on the Wednesday and Friday before your marathon (unless the marathon is on Saturday, in which case shift these days to Tuesday and Thursday).

- The pace of the Tuesday run should be at least 1 minute per mile slower than marathon goal pace and slower if you're still tired from the weekend session. You may also do a few acceleration gliders on this day, but be careful. Never hesitate to slow down on the Tuesday, Wednesday and Friday runs.

- You have some flexibility on the number of minutes to be run during the week. Never increase the amount more than 10 percent above what you have been doing the week before. Don't hesitate to cut back on some of these days if you're feeling tired from the (hopefully) playful but tiring weekend.

"Run/walkers who finish marathons also achieve many other benefits, including weight loss, increased fitness, stress reduction, and group camaraderie. At a time when obesity is epidemic (and a major risk for hypertension, cardiovascular disease, diabetes and some cancers), we should encourage Americans to exercise regardless of athletic ability. Marathon training establishes exercise as a regular part of your life . . . the marathon course has room for everyone —elite runners, joggers, run/walkers, walkers, and wheelchair athletes. Road racing, including the marathon, is like no other sporting event in that the casual athlete can participate in the same event as world-class athletes . . . we are out there to have fun, run injury-free, and improve our health."

–Thomas G. Martin
The Washington Post

MARATHONS ON WHEELS

Several elite wheelchair athletes have told me that they have adapted the schedules and techniques in this book in training for marathons and have improved their times.

II INSPIRATION

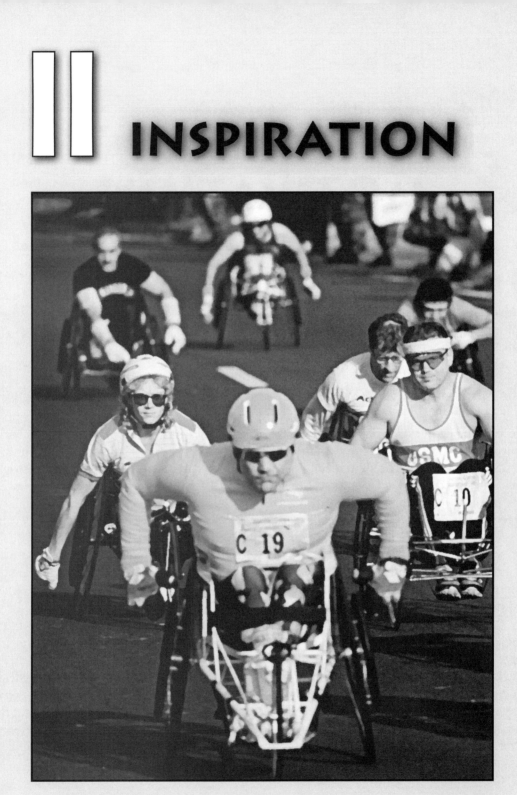

7 THE SOURCE OF MOTIVATION

Just a few minutes each day will keep you motivated and will make you a more positive person. Every year, from hundreds of satisfied marathon finishers, I hear the answer to the question: Why do we take on the challenge of the marathon?

The left brain: logic

Inside the left hemisphere at the top of your head is the center of logic. The left brain solves math problems, organizes and nit-picks, and conducts the structured cognitive activities during your workday. One of the primary missions of the left brain is to steer you in the direction of pleasure and away from discomfort. Any form of stress or perceived stress will stimulate a stream of messages telling you to "slow down!" or "quit!" or to question your sanity: "Why am I doing this?"

Because we rely upon the left side for logical guidance, we listen to these messages. If we're weak or tired, we're very likely to give in to them and compromise our goal. Certainly we must always monitor the real dangers that could produce health problems (heat buildup, traffic, over-fatigue) and take appropriate action.

Most of the time, however, our left brain overreacts, warning us long before we are in real danger. Motivation training desensitizes us to such extraneous messages and the left brain's nagging.

The right brain: intuition

Your creative and intuitive center is in the right side of your brain. Running is one of the best ways to tap into your right brain, as long as you're running slowly enough to stay within your capabilities. This right side is a reservoir of creative solutions to just about any problem, challenge, or obstacle. Through pacing, walk breaks and blood-sugar boosting, you can cut down dramatically on stress, reducing the messages from the left brain so that you stay on the right (brain) track. Later in this section, I'll go over some proven methods of stimulating right brain activity. To maximize time in the wonderful world of the right brain, become sensitive to the stress buildup of your runs and the marathon itself. Only you have the complete power to reduce the intensity and disconnect the negative speaker of the left brain before it makes your running seem like work.

WHY TRAIN FOR A MARATHON?

- "The marathon date on the calendar made me highlight other activities in my life more than ever."

- "I'm a CEO, am financially secure, but nothing in my life has given me the same internal satisfaction as finishing this marathon."

- "Before I started training for the marathon, my friends called me 'Whiner.' Now they address me as 'Captain Confident.' It's true."

- "Once I learned how to pace myself, I got a great attitude boost after every run."

- "The marathon training gave a purpose to my physical side, which I had neglected. I am hooked for life."

- "There is no other activity in life that bestows respect, from inside and from the general population, as training for and finishing a marathon."

- "The day I returned from finishing my first marathon, at age 42, my co-workers and friends had a subtle but definite new respect for me. That has continued for 15 years."

- "Marathon training made me feel like a whole person—body and mind working together as a team."

- "I never imagined that I had the inner strength to go on when stressed until I did my first marathon program. The confidence has allowed me to get a better job, be a better mom, and enjoy myself . . . for being myself."

The motivational track

There are many quick fixes that can get you out of the door or a mile down the road. I actually like to have, as a last resort, some of these "dirty tricks" *(see pp. 89–92)* ready when the primary motivation elements are not working. But it's actually quite easy to stay motivated by expressing the positive thoughts, feelings and momentum you get from your runs. Just a few minutes each day will help you understand the process of staying motivated and will make you a more positive person. In this section you'll find a range of concepts and techniques that have helped thousands of runners to find the spark inside to meet any challenge, starting with the one of rolling out of bed when the alarm goes off.

Getting on the motivational track is as simple as describing out loud for yourself some of the positive things running does for you and others. It may take you a few weeks to set up your motivation routine but, once it is in place, you can stay motivated with a minimum of regular, fine-tuning exercises. You'll learn about developing a vision and how to transform this into a real and satisfying mission. Some quick and simple belief exercises are included to help you mobilize your enjoyment of running and point you toward your mission. All of us have much more potential than we usually allow ourselves to explore. It is my mission in the following chapters to help you tap into your potential so that you can head toward the accomplishment you desire—including getting more enjoyment out of life.

You gotta have fun!

In all this there is a magic ingredient that keeps you motivated in just about any situation. When you find ways to have fun during your run, you open the door for the right brain to take over and work its creative magic. You may start it rolling by reading a funny story before your run, visiting a coffee shop with interesting characters, running with a person or group, going to a favorite trail, exploring new countryside. But, don't stop with my suggestions. The best ones are those that allow you to enjoy running. Anything that makes your run special and interesting should be included in your bag of fun tricks.

Vision and focus

No one stays motivated all of the time. Those who are more successful sometimes seem to be always fired up, but they, too, have down times. By concentrating on the positive aspects of your run, several times a day, you become focused on something

that makes you feel good. It only takes a few seconds every two hours or so and you'll be motivated to get out there and collect your endorphins.

To collect your positive thoughts about running and what makes you feel confident and looking forward to your next run, try "the vision exercise":

THE VISION EXERCISE

I'm looking forward to my run because:

- The physical exertion will feel good.
- My legs want to run.
- The increased blood circulation makes me feel more alive.
- I love the way I feel afterward—relaxed and focused, with a great attitude.
- My family appreciates the way I am after a run.
- It's so great to run in the morning to get the mind and spirit mobilized and focused for the day.
- My afternoon run takes away the stress, getting me ready to enjoy my family.
- During the second half of my run and afterward, I'm high on endorphins.

As you notice changes in yourself, you extend the positive effects into other areas of life. You have a better attitude at home and find yourself enjoying your time with your family much more. Stress isn't as much of a problem. You can deal with problems more directly, and you maintain focus to the finish of your work projects. Everything in your life can be better when you run regularly.

The difference between a dream and a vision

Those who don't spend a few moments a day to stay focused are often guided by dreams and illusions that lead first in one direction, and then another, and then in no direction at all. A dream is not connected to reality. It's easy to dream that you'll run the marathon in less than two hours. Even when dreams are within your capabilities, without a well-structured training program and regular mental contact with your vision, dreams are seldom realized and you set yourself up for disappointment.

In contrast, a *vision* is a series of images that can be molded over several months into a realistic behavioral plan that is put into action every week. In effect, you're a sculptor who molds an elusive image into a series of real experiences that prepare you for and lead you to a goal that is realistic, fulfilling, and engaging.

A vision is a perception of experience that you can prepare for by specific physical and mental exercises. To fulfill a vision, you must chart out the exercises, constantly adjusting and fine-tuning them to make the vision more complete and meaningful. With each adjustment, you get more involved in the process and become more motivated.

DREAMS *VS.* VISIONS

A dream is not connected to reality; it may

- often be a fantasy, like the dreams during sleep
- have no direct connection to your past experience
- be spun out of specific items or experiences that you'd like to have but that are unconnected with current behaviors and/or plan of action

A vision is a series of images that

- give a clear path to the final result including the behaviors
- are directly relevant to behaviors you want to change
- break down the grander goal into a progression of behavioral changes
- give a vision of future behaviors at each step along the way
- start with a recent achievement
- lead you through a progression of improving experiences to the goal behavior
- lay the foundation for the future experience with the eating behaviors, exercise behaviors, etc. that are necessary to make your vision happen or support the transformation
- leave you with a reasonably focused and detailed image of the final behavior —physically, mentally, and spiritually

Transform the vision into a mission

Adding the behavioral elements to your vision is as simple as writing the date of your specific goal on a calendar. But the process often starts weeks or months before. It may be the snapshot of an overweight friend finishing a marathon. "If Suzi can do it, I can too," you say. You enter a marathon and write the date on your kitchen calendar. The mission begins with your first run-walk, a 3-miler. During each long run you will solve new problems, make adjustments and apply the revised vision on the next long run. All the way through the program, you're making your vision more realistic. Wearing a big smile, you keep the mission on track all the way to the finish.

Start with a date on the calendar

The marathon will get your attention and motivate you to do things you haven't done in years. You'll get out of bed an hour early and cover the miles, feeling better for it. After those "bad days" at work, you'll find a way to get on the roads because you have the date of that race scribbled on your kitchen calendar. You're rewarded by getting rid of most of the day's stress. There's something powerful about giving yourself a deadline that pushes you down the road on days when you'd just as soon cut the run short.

Watchwords for your mission

When you truly believe in your vision, you believe in yourself. At the same time, you make the mission easier. Choose the watchwords that support your efforts and add any that will help you believe in the success of the mission.

- I look forward to the creative challenges.
- I have the creativity to find fun in every run — and this fun will increase as I progress.
- I have the resources to realize my vision.
- I will develop increased resources that will help me complete my mission.
- I will develop the discipline to get in all of the runs that are listed.
- I will find a way to dig deeper, to keep going on those few occasions when I don't feel like it.
- I will do what is reasonable to support the goal (eating, sleeping, scheduling, etc.).
- I will look forward to the positive changes inside me through this mission.
- This mission will give me a more positive vision for my future in almost all areas of life.

> "The size of the weekly running group is great because you get a lot of individual attention and form a sense of group unity very quickly. We support each other and look forward to seeing each other every week. I recommend this program and this method to anyone I know who wants to train for a marathon. Those who decide to just 'run all out' instead inevitably seem to drop out of their training and never return to marathon running, but those who take Jeff's advice and method seriously have great successes."

8 GETTING MOTIVATED

Inside of each of us is all the motivation we need to get going and stay motivated.

After six to twelve months of regular exercise, most runners have made the lifestyle adjustments that make exercise a scheduled and important part of the day. Before we get to that point, it's necessary to make an effort to reinforce the regularity of exercise and maintain the daily run or walk as a top priority. Sometimes it's as simple as learning to appreciate the rewards, such as those relaxing endorphins. You've been getting them all along, but you didn't take time to enjoy them.

But everyone will have to find some extra diversions from time to time. Some runners look for different birds or flowers during a run. Others test the winter ice and look forward to the challenge of layering to meet the colder temperatures. The prospect of a dip in the pool or a shower in midrun can get you out of the door and keep you out there when the weather's hot.

Most of those who say they just need a little motivation to get into shape are only dreaming. Yes, they have a dream of being a stronger, firmer, more active person, but the dream is not attached to realistic behavior. Dreams are elusive. An image without a series of weekly workouts will stay, merely, an image. If you really want to change behaviors, believing that you can is only the first step. It is the behavioral vision of moving the legs every other day that changes body shape and improves mental outlook. An idea or image is powerful only if it is practiced, refined, and then changed into a vision of permanent lifestyle fun running.

Confidence in the program

To get motivated, runners at all levels need to feel that each day's workout and the program as a whole is doable. When in doubt, it's always better to err on the side of a less demanding program or one that has flexibility. It also helps to study the program before beginning to determine your level of confidence in the schedule and the designer before you get in over your head.

What about down days? Practically everyone who trains for a marathon has setbacks. You're going to be more motivated to stay on a program if you know that it's possible to add more walk breaks, for example, or to reschedule the long runs. Among marathon runners there's a wide range of abilities and fitness backgrounds, so individuals will progress at different rates, and some schedules don't allow for this. For example, if you're scheduled for a 4-mile continuous run and are dreading it, tell that nagging left brain that you're only going to go 1 or 2 miles and will walk most of it anyway. Most runners who do that end up finishing the 4-miler feeling great. Even if you don't feel up to doing a race but know that it would be a good conditioner for you, talk yourself down to an easier time goal or to merely running the first half of the race. With the pressure off, most racers run the whole race in a surprisingly good time.

> "You never hear anyone say, 'Jeez, I'm sorry I went for that workout.'"
>
> –Bob Anderson

The right group will motivate you

If you can find a group of runners at your ability level in your area, join it. Because the group is waiting for you, you'll roll out of bed on mornings you wouldn't otherwise. The chemistry, fun, and bonding that come out of a group run will have you looking forward to the next run. You'll get as much out of helping others as being pulled along yourself on your "dog days."

If there are no groups in your area and you're having trouble getting out for a run,

put on your running shoes and clothes and call a friend who will talk you out of the door. There is a growing number of online running companions for the same reasons. *(For information on groups in your area, see pp. 194–197.)*

CHOOSE A GROUP THAT

- Is composed of people at your level —not the level you want to reach
- Takes walk breaks from the beginning of all long runs
- Runs at a pace that allows you to finish long runs without breathing so hard that you can't carry on a conversation
- Gives you a feeling of comfort and acceptance
- Meets at a time and place that would fit into your lifestyle

---

Watch your blood sugar levels

You may be just half an energy bar away from motivation. If your exercise time is at midday or later and you feel tired and unmotivated, you may suffer from low blood sugar. Waiting for more than two hours to eat a balanced snack or meal (foods high in sugar make the situation worse) will lower your concentration and motivation. Low blood sugar is a significant stress on your system and causes the left side of your brain to unleash a stream of messages, such as: "You'll feel better tomorrow, take the day off," "You have too much to do," or "You'll feel so much better on the couch." An energy snack, with water, about one hour before exercise, will often silence the left brain and get you off the couch.

Overcoming inertia

Even if you're a dedicated runner, there will be days when the gravity that pulls you back to the bed or couch is much stronger than usual. When you're waffling about going for a run, it helps to read (possibly out loud) a list of benefits that you get from running:

- My attitude is better after every run.
- Stress is released and often completely dissolved.
- Natural body chemicals called endorphins relax the body, reducing or eliminating muscle aches and pains.
- My spirit is engaged, leaving me with feelings of accomplishment, confidence, and strength.
- Body and mind are connected, giving me the confidence that comes with being a more "complete" person.
- My right brain is engaged, energizing my creative and imaginative resources.
- I'm finding connections to hidden inner resources that kick in whenever I'm under stress.

Hot tip!

Crossing a street usually breaks the bond of the couch and signals that you're on your way!

Getting yourself out the door

Anyone can become successful at starting a walk or run by setting up a process similar to getting a model train moving when it is just short of the top of a hill. A few extra pushes or pulls to get the momentum started and you're moving down the road with that same momentum. Those who are successful in getting out of the door regularly spend a little time at the beginning to set up a process with a reward system. After going through the series of steps that gets you going, over and over again, one step will lead automatically to the next one.

Screenplays for bad days

Let's say that it was a bad day at work and you really don't want to run. Your mission, should you choose to accept it, is to get the body in motion using whatever tricks, rewards, etc. are necessary. Here are a couple of simple "scripts" that have helped thousands of folks to get moving —and stay moving until the endorphins start flowing. You'll need to adapt the scripts to your situation and rehearse them over and over, especially when you're going home after work each day. The more you rehearse, even on days when you don't need the motivation, the more likely you will move from one step to the next when you do hit a low.

Scene # 1

You're driving home after a terrible work day; you're hungry and your left brain has a dozen reasons why you shouldn't run.

Action

1. Lie to the left brain, saying "I'm not going to run today. I'll take it easy around the house in some comfortable clothes."

2. You arrive home and immediately put on running shoes and clothes, all the while telling yourself, "I'm not going to run today, just going to be comfortable around here."

3. Eat an energy bar or other energy snack and drink your beverage of choice. (*Hint:* caffeine helps.)

4. Put on some favorite music and read some of the affirmations in this chapter and the last one.

5. Stick your head out of the door to see what the weather is doing and then just step outside.

6. Walk to the edge of the block to see what the neighbors are doing.

7. Cross the street and you're on your way!

Scene # 2

Here's another challenge for many runners: getting out of bed early enough to do the morning run. What do you need to do to get yourself from the bed to the street?

Action

1. Look at your clock the night before. Tell yourself what time you will be getting up. Go through a quick mental rehearsal of yourself hearing the alarm and getting out of bed. Have your clothes laid out so that you can put them on without thinking.

2. The alarm goes off. Without thinking, your feet go on the floor.

3. Without thinking, stand up and head for the kitchen.

4. Prepare your beverage of choice: coffee, tea, juice, smoothie, etc.

5. Sip your beverage and put on clothes —as automatically as possible.

6. Walk out the door, not thinking about running.

7. Walk to the street, not thinking about running.

8. Cross the street and you're on your way!

YOU CAN DO IT, FLO!

"Thought you might like to know that at 63 you are not too old to do a marathon. . . .

Jeff had autographed his book for me, saying 'Flo, you can do it.' He really inspired me and when returning home I decided to start training with Team In Training. I am 63 and completed my first Marathon in the Mayor's Midnight Sun Marathon. At my age there were 699 behind me."

9 STAYING MOTIVATED

A body on the couch wants to stay there. But once a body is in motion, it wants to continue in motion.

WHEN YOU WANT TO STOP

Motivation through forward motion

Just as any motivated runner will have less motivation on some days, everyone reaches plateaus. This chapter is dedicated to helping you continue running when you want to stop. Also included are some of my secrets for staying on a schedule when you have lulls in motivation.

If you start your run slowly enough, it takes only a minute or two to be rewarded by the flow of relaxing endorphins and other attitude-enhancing mental hormones. You may need to walk very often, but moving forward is naturally pleasurable to the body and mind when done at an easy pace.

When you pick a challenge such as a marathon and write the date on your calendar, you're more likely to be motivated on those hot, muggy days or when it's freezing outside. Everyone knows that running 26.2 miles requires preparation. This pulls you out of bed when the temperature outside is in the nineties or 10 degrees below, and it keeps you going when you get the urge to cut the run short.

The more stress you place on yourself, the more discouraging messages you'll receive from the left brain, which will make you want to quit. Ease up, take more walk breaks, and you'll get through most of these "walls." If the weather presents you with too much heat or humidity or you went too fast in the beginning or the middle of the run, it may be too late to do anything but walk. Learn from this, and back off early the next time.

Keep your blood sugar level up

Your preferred blood sugar foods can pull you out of motivational lulls. Everyone will experience a blood sugar crash after about 12 to 15 miles. Take a PowerGel or energy bar with you and eat it (with water). For most runners, that will keep the BSL (and motivation) high. These products also help on short runs if you haven't eaten enough before you set out.

Be sure there is no medical problem

It's extremely rare, but there are a few times when you should not push through barriers. If you have or suspect a medical problem—a stress fracture, cardiovascular stress, heat disease, etc., stop immediately and get help. Even though such problems are very unlikely, it's always better to be safe than sorry. Your ache or pain could indicate significant health risks, so it's always better to quit early and talk to a doctor.

A second type of medical alert pertains to over-training and injury. Some aches and pains are early warning signs of injury or excessive fatigue. Experienced runners become very sensitive to the weak links, those knees, tendons, and muscles that become injured most often. By not trying to push on through an early stage injury—back off early or take an extra day off—you may avoid weeks or months of layoff later.

Tricks for tough or fast runs

Almost every runner has at least one tough run every month. Whether it occurs during a tour around the block or during a 23-miler or speed session, here are my tricks for continuing:

- **Slow down** and allow the body and mind to get a break. Take more walk breaks as needed, take more rest between intervals in a speed session, and start back into the run more slowly. The earlier you make an adjustment, the more you'll be able to salvage from that workout or run.

- **Break up** the remaining distance into segments that you know you can do. Take a walk break (or a shuffle break) every 3 to 5 minutes. You know that you can go another 3 minutes, right? If 3 minutes is too long, try 1 minute. Your run or race is a series of these segments to the finish line.

- **Use distractions.** Look ahead to the next mailbox, stop sign, fast-food restaurant, water stop, etc., and tell yourself that you can take a break there. Make sure the segment is short enough so that you feel confident about getting there.

- **Focus** on the person ahead of the person in front of you. By looking ahead, you can be pulled past the person in front of you if you're running in a group or a race. Stay mentally attached to that person, noting the outfit, the printing, the hat, etc. If you're only looking at details, you'll at least be preoccupying the left brain so that it won't zing you as badly or as often.

- **Use a mantra** *(see the sidebar)*. There are various types of words and phrases that will do more than distract you. Practice these and develop more of your own to put yourself into a positive trance.

- **Don't give up.** If you respond to each thought of quitting with the internal resolve that you are going to finish, you will! Positive mental attitude alone can pull you through many difficult situations.

Mantras for staying motivated

Mantras (phrases you repeat to yourself over and over) will connect you to hidden resources that keep you going when you are tired. The specific words you choose will help to make subconscious and intuitive connections with muscles and your inner resolve. As you learn to tap into the right brain, you'll coin phrases that continue drawing on mental or spiritual resources. The following have been used when under physical and mental stress, but consider them only as a primer. The best ones will be your own, those mantras that relate to your experiences with words that work. Action phrases not only keep you going but also help you perform as you find ways to dig deeper into your resources.

ENCOURAGING MANTRAS

To keep you going

- Feet—stay light and quick, keep moving.
- My legs are strong.
- My heart is pumping better.
- More blood in the muscles
- Lactic acid, go away.
- More oxygen, lungs.
- The strength is in there, I'm feeling it.
- Talk crazy to me, right brain.
- I'm feeling creative—I'm making adjustments.
- I feel comfortable—I'm in control.
- I feel good—I feel strong.
- I'm floating.
- Come to me, endorphins.
- This is fun!

DISTRACTION MANTRAS

To preoccupy your left brain so that it won't send you so many discouraging messages. After saying these over many times, you may be able to shift into the right brain.

- Look at that store, car, building, sign, etc.
- Look at that person, hair, outfit, hat, T-shirt design, etc.
- One more step, one more step
- One more block, telephone pole, stop light, etc.
- Baby steps, baby steps, baby steps

VISION MANTRAS

To help you feel that you're getting where you want to be

- I can see the next mile marker.
- I can feel the pull of the finish line.
- I can feel myself being pulled along by the runners ahead.
- I can feel myself getting stronger.
- I'm pushing through the wall.
- I'm moving at the right pace to finish with strength.

FUNNY MANTRAS

To get you to laugh, which is a right brain activity

- I'm running like a clown, ballerina, football player, stooge.
- Float like an anchor, sting like a sponge.
- Where's the bounce?

CREATIVE MANTRAS

To distract you from your boredom

- I'm building a house, railroad, community, bookcase, etc.
- What type of novel could that person ahead of me have written?
- What type of crime could that person on the sidewalk be plotting?
- What type of movie could be staged here?

When your goal isn't motivating any more

Having gone through more than 150 marathon training programs, I've experienced many motivation letdowns. On most of these, I've rebounded, but on a few, I didn't. Burnout and dropout are mental injuries. If you back off and adjust early, you can avoid major burnout later.

TO GET BEYOND THE MID-GOAL WALL:

- Reduce mileage and cut your running days to three a week. Put a lot of walking into these.

- Run and walk in scenic areas, places that really motivate you to run.

- Schedule a social run with a friend or a group of friends.

- Do anything necessary to add more fun to your program: after-run rewards, special outfits or shoes after specific long runs, and so on.

- Adjust your goal event so that it is more motivating. Stay at a special hotel, get some friends to meet you there, or schedule weekend activities with your family (at events such as the Big Sur Marathon or the Walt Disney World Marathon).

- Sometimes it helps to choose another goal event and adjust your training accordingly.

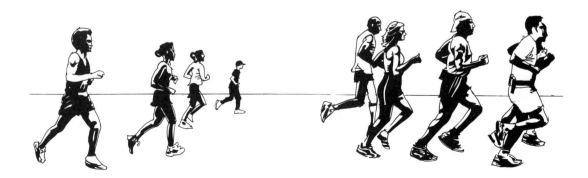

10 THE POWER OF THE GROUP

"I would never have run a marathon if it were not for the group. Looking forward to next year!"

–Moninne Kellaghan, New York City

> You may not be able to find a group, but marathon training will be more fun if you do.

Among those who go through the Galloway Training Program, more than 98 percent complete a marathon. I'm very proud of them, but can't, however, take credit for this rate of success. It's the result of the fun and the bonding that occurs in each pace group as individuals become a team. In a group, individuals who have trouble getting motivated get on track. Competitors who tend to get injured from pushing themselves too hard stay back with the group and stay healthy.

- As a team, you can share the challenges, the laughs, the struggles, and the exhilaration.

- No one needs to go through a tough day without being bolstered by the others.

- As you give support, you'll receive much more in return.

- Every year, in just about every pace group, lifelong friendships are formed.

- Individuals training alone usually reach a plateau of fatigue, injury, lack of motivation, or complications in other areas of life and drop out of the program.

If there is no group in your area, you can start one by running together with just one other person. See the marathon training program flyer at the end of this book. Many lone runners will call friends and talk until they're motivated to get out of the door. Some have simulated group runs by talking on cell phones during runs.

It's interesting to watch the groups develop. On the first day, most are feeling a bit shy, reluctant to say much. After a group run or two, each member develops a sense of belonging and trust. Over the next few months, often without realizing it, each will need to pull at least a little support from teammates, and each will give the same to the others. Through the joking and the gut-level respect generated by meeting challenges together, bonds are established and last a lifetime. Starting as ordinary people, the group will rise to the extraordinary challenge of the marathon.

Some companies are discovering that the power of marathon team-building improves the bottom line as it reduces the waistline. I've seen this experience break down barriers between divisions within a corporation as even the spectators pull for the trainees to meet the challenge. You can't buy the productivity and attitude benefits that come from such a program.

About one-tenth of 1 percent of the population completes a marathon each year. Most individual runners become injured or drop out of their marathon training during the last six weeks. Pace-group programs have almost no dropouts during this same period. Group energy and support creates a bonding and level of respect experienced by few groups in today's world.

Group fun

The most successful groups are those composed of folks at the same conditioning level. The primary goal of the group is to have fun as the distance is covered. I'm not saying that every step is wonderful or every hill bestows joy, but as you exchange jokes and stories and let the chemistry of your personalities create a unique group identity, the fun will emerge.

Homework assignments

If everyone brings a joke, a juicy story, and a controversial issue to every run, group entertainment is guaranteed. Sometimes it takes only one issue, and you can't believe that you're at the end of your run. Take notes on each group run. Bring your disposable camera. There are always a few interesting things that happen, experiences shared, and statements made. Many groups give awards at breakfast after the run: the juiciest story wins a big orange juice.

Keeping the group together

In each of the Galloway training locations, we subdivide the runners into pace groups according to their current conditioning and background. But even in the most evenly matched groupings, one or two individuals will often struggle on each long run. It doesn't hurt a faster runner to slow down: endurance is developed by the distance covered, not the pace. So the group adjusts the pace to accommodate the members who just aren't having a good day.

If someone is huffing and puffing during the first half of the run, slow the pace down at that time, even if the slower person suggests being left behind. During the last 2 to 3 miles, you are going to be huffing, but it shouldn't keep you from carrying on a conversation. If it does, not only does the group need to slow down for the last few miles, but also on the next long run, the pace should be adjusted from the beginning.

Adjusting

During the first few weeks the groups will be a bit fluid, and some of you will want to move up or down. If your group leader suggests that another group's pace would be more comfortable for you, please take the advice. The first priority is that everyone feel comfortable so that the team can stay together. If you're not sure that you're in the correct group, consult your group leader. The best time to change groups, should this be necessary, is during the first three or four weeks, but it's still okay to change after that.

Group rules

- Help the group leader by supporting the walk breaks and keeping the pace slow. Also, help with water, refreshments, etc.

- Everyone in the group should be able to carry on a conversation, even at the end of the run. If anyone is huffing and puffing at all in the first half of the run, slow the pace down and/or take more frequent walk breaks.

- Take all of the walk breaks, early and often. As the long runs get longer, the walk breaks should be taken more frequently. In every group, there are a few macho folks who push for eliminating the first few walk breaks. Hey, these are the most important ones!

- If you're feeling tired (or you sense that someone else is struggling), tell the group leader so that the pace can be slowed.

- When you're feeling great, slow down and stay with the group — don't lead them astray!

- Each member of the group is responsible for his or her own safety. Never assume that others are looking out for you.

- Wear the shirt of your group in case you get separated.

- Keep it fun.

Support your group leaders

It's not an easy job to try to keep everyone in a group from going too fast. On any given run, there are usually one or two individuals who are feeling good and want to increase the pace. By restraining these exuberant individuals at the beginning, the leader will not only help those who aren't feeling good, but also everybody, even the frisky ones, will benefit from the chemistry of keeping the whole group together. Instead of slowing down later and suffering because of the fast early pace, they will all feel strong to the end and will have the best chance of recovering quickly. Don't argue with your group leader when asked to slow down and stay together, even if you think that everybody else must be having a bad hair day or that their blood sugar is low.

Designated sweeper

Even when the pacing is perfect, some individuals may not be able to keep up with the group because of injury or sickness. In each group, each week, a designated sweeper should drop back and stay with that person, providing support or transportation as needed. This assignment will rotate each week. With proper pacing for the group as a whole, this sort of assistance may seldom be needed.

The victory celebration

One of the highlights of our Galloway group training is the celebration after the marathon medals have been won. This gathering is filled with the exuberance of group victory, fun awards, and war stories (some of them actually true). This one event brings together the positive emotions and collective respect into an experience that reinforces the great marathon accomplishment. Be prepared to share stories and to laugh. Just a few of the details, photos, and quotes you collected on the training runs will spice up a great event.

"As I did the Galloway program last year as part of a fundraising effort for the Whitman Walker Clinic in Washington, DC, I combined a great running experience with the feeling of being able to help someone live with HIV/AIDS until hopefully there is a cure. It was my first year of running and the goal was to 'survive' a Marathon. But thanks to the Galloway method, I did more than survive the Marine Corps Marathon—I actually enjoyed running it!

Three things come to mind when I think of the Galloway program:

1) The group experience and the way I looked forward to meeting with 'my' group every Saturday morning and run whatever distance we had to run. I knew I could do it, because there was my group I could rely on and the run-walk method that would keep me going to the last hill.

2) The learning curve from a beginner to a marathoner. I knew I could go the whole distance and did not have to fear 'the wall.' On the contrary, I could look forward to the *exhilarating* feeling of run-walking for hours and still smiling.

3) The hundreds of other runners that we were able to pass during the actual Marine Corps Marathon, because we were still going strong after Mile 15, Mile 18, Mile 23 . . . when other runners slowed down. Thanks to the things we learned during training, I was able to keep my strength all the way to the Finish Line—crossing it with the biggest smile on my face.

Even though I still meet people who do not see the benefits of the Galloway method, I know that the walk breaks will actually help me be faster overall and I will stick to my walk breaks *in order to* reach my time goal!"

–Suzanne Berling

III BREAKING THROUGH

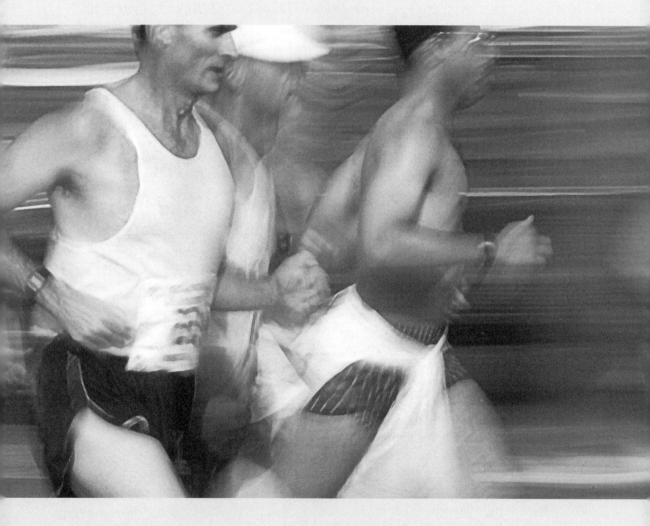

11 A MENTAL TOUR OF THE MARATHON

A thorough mental rehearsal of one of life's challenges will mobilize all of your resources and bring mind and body together.

Before attempting something challenging like a marathon, wouldn't you love to have the confidence of having done it —without the fatigue, sweat, aches, and pains? Thanks to the wonderful world of visualization, this is now possible.

Rehearse!

In this chapter, we're going to rehearse the marathon so that you can immerse yourself in the experience. The better your rehearsal, the more prepared you'll be for the marathon itself. Draw upon your experience from the long runs to construct your mental marathon. The more challenges you rehearse, the less effect they'll have should you encounter them in the marathon itself.

You'll develop a confidence in finishing that is similar to the confidence of veteran marathoners. Even more significant, you'll be gradually adding realistic details and situations to help you overcome the physical and mental challenges of the marathon. This *mental* conditioning will make you tougher and will build the specific confidence you need to confront the same problems in the 26-miler itself. Your long runs help you to desensitize yourself to much of what *could* go wrong.

Benefits of a rehearsal
Familiarity breeds success

Mentally rehearsing the marathon gears up mind and body for the sequence of events. The more times you're able to rehearse, the more smoothly you'll mentally prepare for each segment of the marathon and the better you'll anticipate your need for resources and adjusting for success.

Taking out the garbage

The discouraging messages released under stress are reduced because you've desensitized yourself to them. In other words, there's less stress, therefore less garbage.

Mind and body teamwork

Mental rehearsals are effective practice runs because you can edit and improve responses quickly in your mind. This doesn't get you out of doing your long runs, of course. Once you've had two or three runs over 15 miles, you have an experience base that will allow you to convert 15 minutes of mental rehearsal time into months of training experience.

Taking control

Instead of waiting for things to happen or taking what comes your way, rehearsal allows you to set up the steps you'll take to get through each stage and challenge of the marathon.

Creating the blueprint

Probably the greatest benefit you'll get from rehearsal is the opportunity to mold

---

PRINCIPLES OF MENTAL REHEARSAL

1. **Break down the experience into a series of small events.**
   - None of those events is challenging in itself.
   - Each of them leads directly and automatically to the next.
2. **Desensitize yourself to the uncomfortable parts.**
   - If you have already experienced them mentally, they aren't as bad when you *run* into them.
   - The more you rehearse problems, the more solutions you may find for them.
   - When you mentally "tough it out" in rehearsal, over and over, it's easier to "gut it out" in the marathon itself.
3. **Rehearse every possible "problem" you could have in the marathon itself.**
   - When in doubt, rehearse—it's better to be prepared for anything.
   - Rehearse each problem as if it were worse than you expect it to be in the marathon. Problems that are less intense than rehearsed are less likely to engage the negative left side of the brain.
4. **Rehearse often!**
   - Rehearse parts of the marathon every day.
   - Concentrate on those aspects that make you the most apprehensive.
   - Go through each segment, dealing with each problem and getting through it.
   - You can find several mental solutions to the same problem.
   - At least once a week, do at least a quick mental rehearsal of the marathon, as we are doing now.

your experience in advance, setting up a blueprint for running the marathon. At the same time, you gain insight into the challenges you'll face. Each long run will teach you a few more lessons as it tosses up problems to solve. By the time you've done your 26-mile run, all of the major challenges will have been encountered (except for changes in weather). As you rehearse yourself through the next long run, make the adjustments that you didn't make the last time. The process gets easier and easier even though you're dealing with a greater number of rough edges, components, and anxieties.

Eliminate the negative

The object is not to solve every problem. Many of the doubts, anxieties, aches, and pains just go away as you make a few minor adjustments, dig down a little deeper, and keep going. By rehearsing every possible problem you could have, you'll start the right brain looking for solutions.

Your greatest enemy at any point in the marathon is not the stress. It's the internal doubt your left brain promotes and upon which it feeds. By focusing on magic words and phrases that highlight your past successes, you'll find it easier to ignore the alarmist negativism.

Be creative

As you're being realistic, unleash your creativity. Include in your rehearsal a few unexpected situations that you haven't faced yet. This will reduce your shock and stress if and when these occur in the marathon itself. Be sure to insert some fun rehearsal elements, such as seeing strange people along the way, talking with your fellow travelers, and noticing landmarks. Mental rehearsal will help you to enjoy your marathon.

Let's get mental! Like the real marathon, the mental marathon begins hours before the starting gun goes off.

The night before

First, let's talk through the night before. You've had a full day of walking around the expo, drinking four to six ounces of a sports drink or water each hour, snacking on energy bars and other low-fat and low-salt snacks all day and all evening, and sharing good experiences with friends and with other marathoners from around the country. Now that it's bedtime, what's going through your mind?

- "I'm not going to sleep a wink."
- "It's going to be rough tomorrow."
- "What have I gotten myself into?"

Yes, all of these are legitimate questions. But, the more you frame the marathon as a stressful experience, the more negative messages you'll receive. It's just as easy to frame it as a positively challenging journey.

Get onto that right side of your brain

The left side of your brain has a million logical reasons for why you can't do something. The right side won't try to argue; it will just try to get the job done using its unlimited supply of creative, spontaneous, and imaginative ways of steering you in the direction of your abilities. In most cases, it's easy to switch off the left brain by relaxing, taking the pressure off yourself, and engaging in a right-brain activity, such as laughing, story-telling, or easy physical activity (walking, for example).

Okay, now, what are some positive thoughts about the marathon?

- "Knowing it's over"
- "Having my psychiatrist tell me that I'm okay—even if I want to do a marathon"
- "The satisfaction of finishing with the medal around my neck"

For the first two, your left brain is still in control. Now, concentrate on the medal, the medal around the neck, *that's* the bottom line! Let's start there—you're wearing *your* medal! Sure, there are aches and pains, but overpowering it all is the feeling of accomplishment and personal satisfaction. This is a significant achievement that you accomplished with your own resources. No one can ever take this achievement away.

> This glow will color every other part of the experience. When you start to feel unequal to the task, you'll come back to this very powerful inner feeling that is the result of your finishing.

Warding off the messages

When the left brain bothers you, diffuse the stress by saying that you're not going to push yourself:

- It's going to be a breeze.
- I have all the time in the world to finish.
- This is my day to smell the roses.

Focus on the positive effect of your marathon experience:

- I feel more invigorated.
- The training has improved my attitude.
- My focus is better.

- I'm positive because I'm doing something very positive for myself.

Create a vision of yourself crossing the finish line:

- Sure I'm tired but I'm satisfied.
- The sense of accomplishment is unlike anything I've ever experienced.
- I've found new sources of strength inside.
- The medal around my neck symbolizes all of this—bestows a wonderful glow.

Walk around or jog around:

- The forward motion creates positive momentum.
- My body is designed for forward motion and responds positively when I move.
- Natural endorphins relax me and settle me down.
- This gets the right brain connected to the body, allowing me to bypass the left brain.

Tell a joke:

- Laughing helps to engage the right brain.
- It bestows a gutteral confidence.
- Collect a few funny thoughts and jokes that I can call up with a key word.
- Even if I tell a joke to myself, I can laugh.

Have a number of positive success stories:

- The best ones are the many little successes I've had in marathon training.
- I can also draw from the success stories of others.
- I can trade stories with other runners.
- Positive behavioral experiences build a positive attitude and inspire positive behavior.

You can, and should, use all these techniques in the marathon itself. But, you need to rehearse them before you really need them. Create the scene in your imagination, bring on the star (you yourself!) and watch the scene unfold, with all the lines and all the action. Then play it again, frequently, until you are word perfect—even under stress.

The night before

Yes, you're nervous, but it's normal to feel this way. You may be so nervous that you won't sleep at all. That's also okay because you don't need to sleep the night before a marathon. The crucial nights are the two before the last one. Sleep deprivation may be a good thing when it's limited. Many marathoners, including some world-class performers, have run their best times after a sleepless night. It's not the lack of sleep that is of concern, it's the worrying about not sleeping the night before.

So you're resting, thinking about all of the things that are about to happen to you. You may decide to read or you may just lie there resting. If it's an out-of-town marathon, be sure to bring a magazine, book or something that can keep your interest in those hours of darkness. Positive, interesting concepts or stories are best, but anything that has worked in the past is fine. I bring along the newspapers that pile up on my doorstep between trips.

Wake-up call

Now imagine yourself waking up—you probably got some sleep. You're motivated to get going and begin a water-drinking routine: four to six ounces every half hour. As you collect the items on your checklist,

you develop a vision of the positive, successful feeling you're going to have with the medal around your neck. When the negative side of your brain starts to send its messages, think of the medal around your neck and move into some productive activity.

The line up

It helps to know, in advance, about the starting area, how you'll get there, the problems, etc. In New York City, for example, you must board a bus quite early and sit under a tent for several hours. At the Marine Corps Marathon, you will be walking or taking the Metro to the start, in all probability, and it's a fairly long walk.

Imagine yourself joking with friends or folks as you walk to your starting position and wait for the gun. You've spent a little time preparing for this with some interesting stories and jokes, which you will be sharing. As you're laughing, you realize that the left brain is kept under control and can't unload many negative thoughts.

It's natural to feel nervous and to be excited, so imagine those feelings. Then settle yourself down by saying things such as "I feel relaxed and ready to glide" and "I've prepared and have plenty of power." When you receive even the hint of a left brain message (and you will), squelch it with a positive behavioral thought, such as the vision of yourself going across the finish line. Take a few jogging steps as you mentally rehearse those good thoughts.

The start

Now, rehearse the start. You begin to get uneasy when the announcer calls everyone. But, as you share energy with the people around you, tell jokes, or mentally revisit some very successful experiences, you're feeling comfortable and secure. Stay with that and then watch yourself as the gun fires and you gently move with the people around you. You're all in this together, moving forward toward a positive goal. It's a mass migration in which you're destined to triumph!

Even in rehearsal you'll be tempted, at times, to go faster, to express a few hidden, competitive urges (which you may not know you have). But you hold back. Realizing there is plenty of time and distance to run the pace you wish, the first few congested miles don't bother you as you continue to go with the flow. Several times you find yourself feeling good and starting to run faster than you're ready to run so you return to a realistic pace (or better, a conservative one).

Pushed forward by your left brain ego, you're tempted to not take the first few walk breaks. But at each place for a walk break, you walk. As people go by, and you're tempted to cut the break short, you resist the temptation. Soon you're into the flow of the breaks—mentally segmenting the distance.

> In the real marathon you won't have to imagine the left brain trying to send a stress message about how far you have left to the finish, but in rehearsal you should imagine your response: You immediately focus on your next walk break, saying out loud "Just *x* more minutes before my next walk break."

Imagine yourself walking a minute every mile. After a few miles you'll make it a game to focus on a few individuals who are running at your desired pace. You follow them with your mind's eye as they get ahead on your walk breaks, and as you playfully catch up with them by the end of each running segment. By the 15-mile point, you'll have to choose another set of people because your original group has dropped off the pace by running continuously.

Challenges

It is better to know the course you will be running (study the specific course descriptions in the race flyers). But if you're unsure of the exact route, you can rehearse a generic marathon. It's even better to over-rehearse the challenges; if you're prepared for a more difficult experience, a less demanding one won't engage the left brain as much.

Hills present a variety of challenges. In the early stages, you may have a tendency to run a bit too hard going up so you hold yourself back. When you reach a difficult uphill, a slight shortening of the stride will relax the legs again and keep you moving with strength. When hills get difficult later on, you continue to shorten the stride, even as short as tiny "baby steps," if needed. This allows you to keep moving and get the job done. It's always better to rehearse hills that are longer, steeper and more frequent than those actually on the course.

The most significant challenges will come during the last 6 miles when the left brain is going to be activated by a variety of stresses: fatigue, blisters, aches, fatigue, low blood sugar, dehydration, *fatigue*. If you over-rehearse the difficulty of the last six miles of the marathon, you'll be in a better position to enjoy the end of the marathon itself.

Gutting it out

Most of the problems, insecurities, and resulting negative messages can be managed and overcome by digging down a little deeper into your reservoir of fortitude. This source of strength comes directly from your spirit, which has the capacity to generate positive momentum continuously. By rehearsing yourself through the low points, you not only become stronger but also develop the intuitive paths that can connect you to these resources in the future: for fitness, work, personal challenges, and other areas of life.

On to the finish

And so we end where we began. The positive flow of energy toward the finish line is your destiny, pulling you past the challenges, through the doubts, and out of the depths of uncertainty itself. You've done this yourself, and you've developed a lot more than physical capabilities along the way. That medal symbolizes a significant internal journey that has unlocked treasures that will continue to enrich you.

"I recently ran my first marathon doing all the wrong things and I have to thank you for your help. I was at a surgeons' convention at San Diego June 2 and they were having their Rock and Roll Marathon. The longest I had run was 8 miles and the most mileage I ran weekly was 25. I weigh 210, and am 45 years old but what the heck, I decided to go as far as I could. At 6 miles this group passed me following a pacer with a 5 hour sign. Wow!!! I decided to follow them and to my surprise they started to walk and I was told it was *your* technique!!!! I was dead tired with my new shoes and cramps at the last 2 miles but I *finished* at 4:59:14."

–Ignacio Echenique, M.D.

12 MAGIC MARATHON WORDS

Magic words distract you from the discomfort, while they lead directly to the extra horsepower that all of us have hidden inside.

By using a few special words, you can pull yourself out of the slump in motivation and physical energy that usually happens at some point during long runs. I've heard from several runners who, when the fatigue settled in, started to feel sorry for themselves and slow down but then, through a liberal use of magic words, ran a personal record or close to it. Even when your conditioning and the weather conditions stop you from a fast performance, the use of these words can mentally reframe any experience into a positive one.

Magic words give you another means of taking control of your performance. They allow access to the internal patterns of dealing with stress and pulling up hidden strength. I like to compare this network of inner connections to a mass of tangled wires, some making strength connections, some going to insecurity and negativity, and a lot of loose ends. You train yourself to make the right connections to stay positive, deal with real problems, and pull the strength available when needed. Called

positive reinforcement, this technique is the same as that described as "brainwashing," except reversed.

Positive brainwashing

My three magic words are **relax**, **power**, and **glide**. I started using them during my competitive career to deal with three problems I encountered during difficult runs and races.

Relax

Usually at the end of a hard run, when I feel my resources slipping away, I have a tendency to tense up because I think that things are going to get worse. I used to slow down and obey the stream of negative messages. Now, I know that the left brain is really bluffing, making conditions seem much worse than they really are. When I feel the first sensation of tightening, I focus on pushing beyond the stress by saying the word "relax" to myself. After two decades of use, I can now feel an instant, subtle relaxation.

Power

When I start slowing down, the left brain tells me my strength is almost gone and issues a warning "You may not finish," or "Stop now before it gets worse." As soon as I say the word "power," I feel my strength rebuilding and am reassured that everything is going to be all right.

Glide

During the latter stages of any long or hard run, my form gets shaky. To counter this trend, I say the word "glide" and instantly I feel smoother (even when I don't look any smoother). I've now associated this magic word with hundreds of runs when I started to get the "wobbles" but finished with a feeling of good form and efficiency. Now, when I say "glide," I'll receive a bit of the same sensation I felt at the end of some of my best lifetime efforts, although my pace is sometimes twice as slow.

> To remember this, think "R–P–G" as you run.

When you say the magic words:

- You instantly feel in control.
- The words at first confuse and distract the left brain, cutting off the negative messages for a while.
- A surge of confidence builds as you apply the words.
- Positive memories flood the subconscious and sometimes the conscious, further cutting out the left brain.
- Sometimes this series of events will jump-start the right brain, helping you find intuitive solutions to current problems.

- You relive (and are energized by) the past experiences where you started to lose it but were able to refocus on the positive.
- On a few occasions, you may set a personal record, finish an impossible run, or pass a competitor you haven't beaten before.
- More likely, you'll be able to complete the run you were capable of running on that day.
- With each use, you become more confident and effective in using your own magic.

Making your words magic

As in any program, you must have a continual training regime to develop and fine-tune these responses. The words aren't magic in themselves. They come alive and make better connections as you associate each with experiences in which you overcame specific problems. The more experiences, the more magic.

1. Start by listing the problem areas for which you could use some inner strength: relaxation, motivation, continuing under adversity, digging deeper.

2. Go back in your memory bank and list, beside each problem area, as many specific instances as possible in which you overcame the problem.

3. Attach a key word or phrase to each experience. The more experiences you have catalogued under one of these keys, the more powerful their effect.

4. Each time you overcome one of these problems again, add a new experience to the category and attach the key word to it.

As you add more experiences, the magic of the words becomes more powerful. You're training your mind to set in motion the same complex set of reactions that produced the success in the past. Intuitively, you also set in motion a search for the many little connections inside that give you a feeling of control and power.

Use these as needed to take off the pressure and bring back the confidence. Add more key words and the accompanying thoughts that make sense to you. Subtract items that don't engage you. You are molding this to fit your needs like a glove.

> **Hot Tip:** Photocopy this and the next page and read during your walk breaks.

The magic thoughts

Relax

- There's no pressure on me; I'm here to have fun.
- I'm going slowly. If it gets tough, I'll just slow down more.
- From the first step, I'm going to relax and enjoy the endorphins.
- I feel comfortable, supported by all this energy.
- I'm part of a very positive movement.

Power

- I feel good about myself and what I'm doing.
- This experience gives me control over myself.
- I know what I'm doing when I'm out here.
- This is my heritage; the power of the human migration spirit is with me.

Achievement

- I've developed great self-respect through this marathon and the training.
- I created this level of fitness, and I'm very proud of it.
- Each step is producing benefits.
- This achievement builds upon a long series of successes.

I'm storing energy

- I've got all day—enjoy!
- Slow down and savor this moment.
- I'm going to store this energy away.

Walking extends resources

- The walk breaks push back my wall.
- Every person who passes me is pulling me along.
- This side of the road is my walk break lane; I own it.
- Walk breaks give me power.
- Walk breaks are my heritage.
- I only have x more minutes (until the next walk break).
- Walk breaks hold back the energy tide so it will surge at the end.

No problems will get to me

- I've got all the resources I need.
- Everyone feels discomfort.
- I'm hanging in there.
- I'm working through this.
- The problem is easing; it's going away.
- I can slow down and feel better.
- I can shorten my stride and relax the muscles.

Muscles, listen to me!

- I'm shortening stride and shuffling.
- Movement pulls out the cramp.
- The muscle is loosening up.

I love hills!

- I have the power to zoom up this hill, but I'm going to save it.
- I'll shorten stride down to "baby steps," if needed.
- I'm low to the ground and feeling light on my feet.
- My muscles are relaxing; I've got the strength.
- The hill is working with me to pull me up.

Short (stride) is better

- I'm shortening stride and feeling more power.
- Just a little stride shortening makes the muscles relax.
- This shorter stride gives me more control.
- With a shorter stride, I can turn over my legs better.

I'm getting there!

- I'm tired but strong.
- I'm feeling better.
- I'm tired but proud.

- There's plenty of strength left.
- The reward is coming.
- What wonderful accomplishment!
- Fewer than one-tenth of 1 percent of the population can do this—and I'm doing it!
- Tight legs are a sign of accomplishment; I'll shorten my stride and run smoothly.

Don't lose the magic

Some runners can get a quick fix by using the word "power," for example, to pick up the pace for a hundred meters or so in the middle of a race. This will almost always lead to a significant slowdown at the end of the run.

Magic words gradually program your internal systems to pull together in an instant the complex series of internal connections that produced success in past experiences. Invoking an isolated word to dramatically turn around the natural effects of fatigue can increase speed for a short distance, but will use up valuable resources you need in the long run.

You don't have to give in to any negative message that hits you when you're under stress. By focusing on the positive, you maintain control. It's what you put in the forefront of your thoughts that counts.

TWO MILESTONES

"The milestone of turning 50 in June 2000 was the motivation for my joining the Galloway Marathon training. It turned out to be the most memorable present I could have given myself. I had never run but was always a 2-mile walker. I wanted to prove to myself that I was 'on top of hill —not over it.' In December, the feeling of crossing the finish line at the Jacksonville Marathon will live with me forever. I was even first in my age division—granted there were only three women in my age group, but I was #1!!!!! It may have taken over 6 hours, but I achieved my goal. I finished and was ready to celebrate yet another milestone—my Marathon at 50 Milestone!"

–Nancy Homan

13 DIRTY TRICKS

"When I was feeling at the end of my resources, at mile 24, I tried one of your dirty mental tricks. It gave me a sense of control, and I ran the last mile with a smile on my face."

A really good rehearsal (with good pace judgment) will pay off by pulling you most of the way through the marathon. By adding your magic words, you'll push on for 2, possibly 5, miles further, sometimes all the way to the finish line. But there are moments in every marathon, usually near the end, when the magic seems to have gone out of your words, and worse, your legs. This opens up a big microphone into which the left brain shouts its messages. You've probably heard most of them:

- "It's over. Just walk to the finish."
- "Slow down; it'll feel much better."
- "Stop now and feel great."
- "Oh, do I feel bad."
- "I can't do it today."
- (And the worst one of all) "Why am I doing this?"

Dirty tricks as distractions It's time to play some dirty tricks on your left brain, After all, it does the same to you all the time. Almost anyone gets these messages. You're only in trouble if you listen to them. Dirty tricks distract the left brain so that you

can get further down the road. But they can do so much more. As you find a series of creative images that get you into your right brain, you'll trigger other imaginative thoughts. These may entertain you, but they are most effective when they jump-start right-brain activity, which produces intuitive solutions to problems.

When you get it working, the right brain acts like a hacker trying to break through Pentagon security codes. It keeps probing, hitting dead ends, and trying again until it finds the direct connections to the centers that get the job done. In addition, right-brain activity improves motivation and keeps your organism working all the way to the finish.

If you've trained according to the schedules in this book and pace yourself realistically in the marathon itself, you will be, physically, on the express train to the finish. There is, however, a very real mental wall that most marathoners must push through to get within sight of the finish line. By doing your mental training, you'll push the wall back closer and closer to the finish.

Mental rehearsal

If you've really immersed yourself in regular and effective mental marathon rehearsals for at least twelve weeks leading up to the marathon, you'll cruise through most of the problem areas during the first 18 to 20 miles. An increasingly effective mental rehearsal *(see pp. 78–84)* will keep you on track and off the beam of the negative left brain for most of the marathon.

Magic marathon words

After the mental rehearsal loses its effectiveness and stress causes the negative messages to increase, it's time for some magic words *(see pp. 85–88)*. By attaching an increasing number of successful experiences to your magic marathon words, you can flood the brain with positive memories and renew the subconscious performance connections that got the job done before. This positive brainwashing will usually push back the mental wall to the 23- to 25-mile mark.

Shifting into right brain gear Just as overall physical fatigue is delayed by regular shifts in running form, mental freshness is maintained by shifts back and forth between the left and right brain. Mental strength is developed through rehearsal and use of your magic words. As you find it easier to shift into the right brain, you'll delay even further the point where your attitude won't respond.

Dirty tricks are reserved for that aggravating place, late in the marathon, when a growing stream of mental e-mail bombs from the left brain are invading and attacking your will to go on. As you find a series of creative images that activate the right brain, you will trigger other imaginative thoughts to keep you exercising to capacity all the way to the finish line. *Dirty tricks are merely crazy ideas that can't be grasped by the left brain because they are not logical.* Let's go through one of these so that you can see the dynamic aspects of their effects.

Subverting the left brain

Trying to overwhelm the left brain with distracting left-brain activity doesn't work. Some folks try to counter the discouragement of left-brain activity with logical challenges. For example, to counter the message "This marathon is going to hurt," some will mentally work on a math problem or construct some business situation or analytical exercise.

This may distract your left brain for a while and keep its demoralizing messages at bay, but your thoughts are still under its control. It is only a matter of time until a major or continuous stress wave will overwhelm this temporary distraction. When your stream of mental messages is hooked to the left hemisphere, you'll tend to get increasingly more persistent messages of a negative nature.

The greatest drawback of this approach is that you lose the intuitive capacity to reach toward high goals. By shifting into the right side of your brain, you have the opportunity to search for hidden strengths and find spontaneous motivation, inspiration and even entertainment that you didn't know were there.

Sneak down the road while the left brain is confused

Conjure up an image that the left brain, with all of its logic, doesn't know what to do with. While it is befuddled, you have a window of opportunity to block out negative messages and move toward your goal. The more you elaborate on and fill out the scenario of the dirty trick, the more time you'll have before the negative side starts broadcasting discouragement again. You may get 100, 200, or 400 meters down the road. But the finish line is only a series of dirty tricks away.

One crazy thought can unlock another

Even one imaginative dirty trick can start the creative side of the brain working on other interesting images, visions, and notions that will entertain you and get you closer to the finish. More significantly, a series of these tricks can unlock the creative process inside you and mobilize all of your resources in overcoming challenges and getting you to the finish line feeling good.

The best dirty tricks are those that work for you. Only you will respond to the unique chemistry of specific images and crazy concepts. Start concocting these during your right-brain runs and remember the ones that work. The more you use them, the more effective they become.

A bag of dirty tricks

Almost any imaginative idea will distract you for a while. To engage the performance components inside, it helps if the tricks are related to behaviors that help you in the marathon. Here are a few ideas that have worked for me.

The giant invisible rubber band

On all marathons, I carry with me this device, which is mounted to my shorts in the small of my back. When someone passes me in the late stages, my left brain explodes with a stream of discouragement: "Look how smoothly he or she is

running, and how ragged you are." It's easy to listen and give in to those logical messages, which are only trying to reduce my effort and slow me down.

Instead, I attack by throwing the giant rubber band over the head of whoever had the audacity to pass me. For a while, the lead may grow. During the next few hundred meters, I fill in a great number of details, such as imagining how the tension on the rubber band is increasing and cutting off the oxygen supply to the brain of the person I have "rubber banded." Surely he or she will have to slow down.

At some point I must laugh at myself for such a ridiculous conception. But laughing helps to send me into the right side of my brain, and I relax. Limber legs turn over quicker, and I usually catch up with, or pass, the person who passed me. The giant invisible rubber band has worked again!

Oxygen molecules

The night before a marathon, I pretend to collect several million oxygen molecules in a sandwich bag, which I pin onto my shorts. During the latter stages of the marathon, when the oxygen doesn't seem to be as abundant, I take off the bag and squeeze it out in front of my mouth or nose. Before squeezing, I exhale every third or fourth breath completely. Just one or two squeezes will last about 100 to 200 meters. The best part of this trick is seeing and hearing the reactions from the people around me in the marathon. If you're a real salesperson, you may try to make some money from those folks who went out too fast and are now severely oxygen-deprived. Just bring along some extra bags.

Ball-bearing atoms

This is a high-tech right-brain invention that will send you gliding to the finish. As the legs lose their resilience near the finish, you can shake off from your hair millions of atoms that normally act to keep it shiny. As the atoms drop onto your feet, you'll find that you don't need to stretch out your stride any more. You glide better through the air and stay more efficient by staying closer to the ground. When you're losing this effect, shake your hair again. Balding people, like myself, will always appreciate some strategic head shakes from others. A downhill portion of the course will enhance the effect of these virtually invisible ball bearings.

The giant hand

The ancient Greeks often imagined that Zeus or another god was helping them. When it becomes tough to go up a hill during those last 6 miles, call for the giant hand to come in and gently push you up. Most folks find that the hand comes in gently as you straighten up your posture. The support increases as you shorten stride, keep feet low to the ground, and let the feet gently lift off when they are directly underneath you.

Your "inspiration" shoes

If logistics permit, you might consider changing shoes during the last 6 miles of the marathon. Both pairs must be broken in, of course. Save your "inspirational" pair for the last part. Just putting them on sends a jolt of invigoration into your feet, up your legs, then through your body and into the right brain. At that point, all types of crazy and innovative things can happen.

The extra-special energy bar

For the marathon journey, you're not bringing just any energy bar. You spent some time the day before picking the ones with the greatest energy potential and you infused them with even more energy. Handle the pieces of these bars with care as you don't want to infuse everyone around you. As you chew on each piece and drink water, you feel the energy move from your mouth to your right brain. Then, instantly it unlocks other pockets of energy that have been hidden until now.

Have fun with these dirty tricks. Since your only constraint is the imaginative power of your right brain, there are no limits to what you can conjure up and unleash when needed.

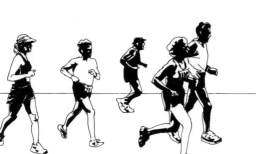
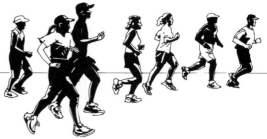

IV THE BIG DAY

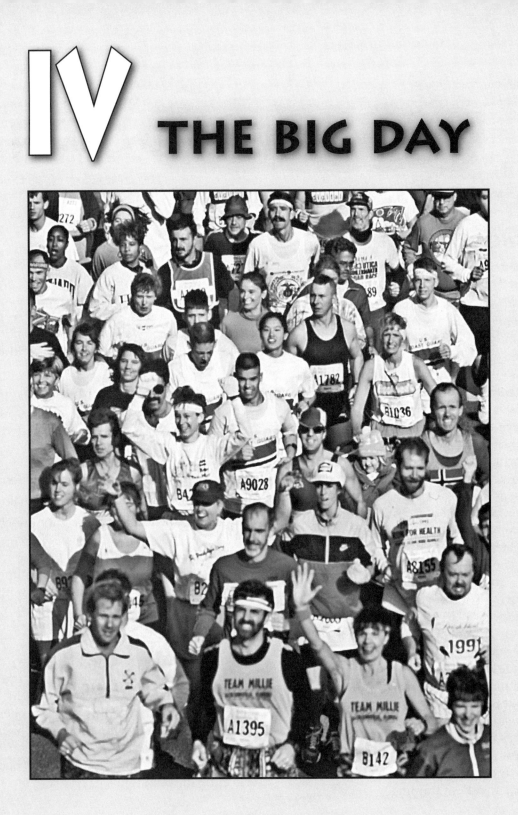

14 COUNTDOWN

TWO DAYS TO THE RACE

You can still improve your performance in the last 48 hours

Although the physical training has been done, you can, in the last two days, significantly enhance the way you feel afterward and the quality of your performance by choosing certain behaviors and avoiding others. Graduation day is near; don't let your vision get cloudy. You can still improve your performance during the last 48 hours.

Because of nervousness, the excitement of the expo, and the distractions of another city, the marathon, friends, and so on, it's easy to lose concentration on a few key items. Be sure to read this section over several times during the last few weeks so that you're more likely to keep the mind and body on track.

You need to be in charge of yourself during the crucial 48 hours before the marathon. In this way you can control your attitude, your eating, your schedule, and so on. This doesn't mean that you should stay by yourself in a hotel room eating salt-free pretzels and energy bars and drinking water. Being with friends is positive. You have veto power over what goes into your mouth, where you go, and how late you stay out. Being in control of your destiny is the primary step in running faster without training.

Be positive

Have a list of statements, similar to the Magic Marathon Words, that you can repeat as necessary. You're going to have discouraging thoughts slipping out from the left brain so we'll work on a way to bypass them and move into the world of the positive.

- I have no pressure on myself.
- I'm going to enjoy this.
- I'll start very slowly.
- The people are great.
- Because I started slowly, I'm finishing strong.
- The satisfaction of doing this is unequaled.
- I've developed a great respect for myself.

Drink!

During the 48 hours before the marathon, drink at least four to six ounces of water every hour you're awake. If you're sweating, drink more. If you prefer to drink juices or electrolyte beverages, then do so. Try to avoid drinking too great a quantity of fluids that are loaded with sugar. Even apple juice and orange juice have a high sugar content so take this into consideration as you watch your blood sugar level. Your best defense against dehydration is to drink water continuously until you hear sloshing in your stomach.

Avoid the dehydrating elements

Alcohol

During the 48 hours before the marathon, it's best to avoid alcohol completely. Your exercising muscles and kidneys will thank you.

Caffeine

For those who dearly love their cup of coffee on race morning, go ahead. But make it just one cup, and drink a glass of water before the coffee and at least one glass of water afterward.

Salt

This is probably the leading cause of dehydration for most marathoners. Because it's used so widely in most restaurants, you're likely to consume large amounts of salt, without realizing it, when you're away from home. For this reason:

- Try to avoid restaurant food during the 24 hours before the marathon.
- Eat foods that you know do not contain salt (or are very low in salt).
- Drink a little more water than normal if you've consumed food that may have some salt in it.

Even one salty meal the night before a marathon will leave you significantly dehydrated for the marathon itself—no matter how much water you drink. So if you go to the pasta-loading party the night before, watch out for the sauce and the garlic bread! (Just nibble on the pasta and digest the conversation.)

Medications

Most medications (especially those for colds, flu, and the like) have a dehydrating effect. Be sure to consult with a doctor who is aware of the various effects of running on the body and have your medication adjusted accordingly.

Eat!

The best eating plan for the 48-hour marathon countdown is the best eating plan for life in general: keep eating low- or non-fat snacks continually, all day long. Avoid eating a large, heavy meal in the afternoon or evening before the marathon. If you want to snack on energy bars all afternoon or have a series of carbohydrate snacks that you know will get through your system quickly, do so. Concentrated forms of sugar (frozen yogurt, syrup, and candy) are not recommended.

Check out the staging area

If it is possible, go over the staging area the day before. As a guide, you can't beat someone who has run that marathon before: he or she will know where you'll be arriving, where you can keep warm and relax, and the best way to get to the portion of the road where you'll be lining up. If you get a clear idea of all this ahead of time, you'll feel more in control and will tend to receive fewer messages from the left brain.

Rest

You don't have to sleep, but you must rest. Settle into your home or hotel room and relax in the best way you know. Read, watch TV, listen to music, talk with friends, but relax. Again, take control of your environment and mold for yourself a positive and cozy atmosphere. Don't worry if you don't sleep at all, but lay that head down and store up some energy.

Wake up

Set your wake-up call so that you have plenty of time to get moving, gather your gear together, and go through the eating and drinking timetable that worked for you during the long runs.

Follow your drinking plan

Drink a glass of water after you wake up. Cut off water intake as you do before long runs, and use the bathroom before the start of the race (limiting stops during the race).

Eat before you start

A snack before running will hold your blood sugar level up for the first half of the marathon. One of the reasons I've advocated eating before all of your long runs is to have the opportunity to discover the foods and the pattern of eating that will work best for you in the marathon itself. About 70 percent of those in our various training groups find that energy bars are digested most quickly and provide the best blood-sugar stabilizing effect. You should use what has worked best for you in your food countdown before long runs. Eating about 200 to 250 calories of high-quality carbohydrates about an hour before a run has helped many runners to keep their blood sugar level stable for the first half of the marathon—but use what worked for you in training.

Start slowly

Almost everyone who performs a personal record in the marathon runs the second half faster than the first. Slow down by 10 to 20 seconds per mile (from your projected marathon pace) during the first 3 to 5 miles, and then follow the guidelines on the pace chart on p. 189. Many marathoners report that, by starting out 15 seconds per mile slower, they have the resilience to run 20 to 30 seconds per mile faster at the end of the marathon.

Take walk breaks

A high percentage of those who didn't achieve the time goal they desired in the marathon when they were running continuously have been able to improve their finishing times significantly by walking *(see pp. 14–22 for walk break suggestions on race day based on goal pace)* from the beginning of the marathon.

Eat while running

Small carbohydrate snacks eaten during the second half of the marathon with a cup of water have helped marathoners improve their time goals by boosting their blood sugar levels. This maintains mental concentration, sustains a positive mental attitude, and reduces the opportunity for negative messages from the left brain to creep in. Be sure to reread part VI, "Food and Fat Burning," and especially chapter 22 —"Boosting Blood Sugar and Motivation." Don't try anything new, unless you've never tried any blood-sugar-boosting food during long runs. In this case, hard candies or gummy bears will safely boost blood sugar with little chance of problems.

Pacing tips for the marathon

For the first 3 to 5 miles:

- Run at marathon pace during the running parts and take the walk breaks.
- For the average person, a 1-minute walk break will slow you by 10 to 15 seconds.

- A slightly slower pace will allow the legs to warm up before they are pushed into race effort.
- Remember to adjust your pace for heat, humidity, and hills.

Between 3 and 8 miles:

- Run faster in the running portions *and* take the walk breaks.
- You will gradually pick up the pace so that by 8 miles, you're running at goal pace when you average out the walk breaks and the running segments.
- If it's a struggle to pick up the pace, maintain a level of effort that is comfortable.
- Don't even think about cutting your walk breaks short to speed things up.

Between 8 and 18 miles:

- Run at marathon goal pace (running faster to compensate for walk breaks).
- Stay smooth as you ease down to walking and ease back into running.
- Compute your pace each mile. Uphill miles can be slower, and downhill miles can be faster than your goal pace.

After 18 miles:

- You can cut out the walk breaks if you're feeling strong (and want to) or, for several walk breaks, walk for only 30 seconds, and then eliminate them entirely.
- If you need the breaks but your legs are cramping, shuffle instead of walking (feet low to the ground—light touch).

After 23 miles:

- You can keep picking up the pace if you feel up to it.

HAVE FUN!

By staying within your physical capabilities from the beginning, you can enjoy the people, the joking, the sights, and the overall experience. Be gentle on yourself throughout the marathon and the enjoyment will flow. For sharing purposes, don't forget to bring with you a joke, an interesting story, a controversial issue, and/or some gossip. Of course, bring along anything else like this that doesn't weigh much and will add to the fun.

Marathon day checklists

In general

- Drink four to six ounces of water every hour.
- Mentally rehearse the marathon, feeling good, overcoming challenges, recovering.
- Eat small carbohydrate snacks constantly.
- Relax with friends or family.

The night before

- Drink four to six ounces of water every hour as long as you are awake.
- Eat light carbohydrate snacks such as energy bars.
- Relax, laugh, enjoy the moment.
- Go over the procedure, route, and so on for getting to the start.
- Do a very relaxed mental rehearsal of the marathon, concentrating on the positive.
- Pack your bag.

Your marathon bag should contain:

- Race number and pins
- Race instructions, map, etc.
- A copy of The Marathon Morning List *(below)* and a copy of Magic Marathon Words *(see pp. 85–88)*
- Shoes, socks, shirt, shorts, and warm-up suit
- Other clothes if it's cold: tights, polypro top, long-sleeved T-shirt, gloves, hat, ear covering, etc.
- Water (about 32 to 64 ounces)
- Bandages (Second Skin is excellent), Vaseline, etc.
- $20–$30 in cash (for transit fees, etc.)
- energy bars or your chosen carbohydrate source (enough for the start, for the second half, and for after the marathon)
- A fanny pack or plastic bags, safety pins
- Some extra shirts and/or pants as extra layers in case the staging area is cold; be prepared to leave them behind when you begin the marathon.
- Garbage bags as an inexpensive waterproof top and ground cover
- Prepare to bring a controversial issue, an interesting story, and a few jokes.

To do on marathon morning

- Drink as you did before long runs.
- Eat—according to the schedule that has worked for you before the long runs. For example: one energy bar with eight ounces water, one to two hours before the start.
- Bring your bag, car keys, etc.
- Leave at least 30 minutes before you think you'll need to leave, in case of traffic.

- If you have to spend several hours at the race site before the start, stay warm, get off your feet, and relax. Bring a newspaper to read and/or sit on.
- An hour before the start, walk around the staging area to mentally rehearse yourself lining up.
- A half hour before the start, walk around for 15 minutes to get the legs moving.
- Jog for between three and five minutes (very slowly) just before lining up.
- Keep the legs moving, in place if necessary, as you stand waiting for the start.
- If you are going for a time goal, get to the starting area early enough to secure a good place.
- If your goal is, as it is with most of us, "to finish," you should line up in the back of the crowd.
- Joke around and enjoy the energy and personalities of the folks nearby.
- Go out slowly. If it's hot, go out even more slowly!
- Get over to the side of the road and take *every* walk break, from the beginning. Each walk break gives you a chance to appreciate and enjoy each mile.
- Drink at *every* water station until you hear sloshing in your stomach.
- Slow down by 30 seconds per mile for every 5°F temperature increase above 60°F.
- If you feel warm, pour water over your head at each water stop.
- When you get tired, shorten your stride.
- Don't stretch during the run or immediately afterward.
- You may cut out the walk breaks after mile 18 if you're feeling good.

Immediately afterward

- Grab water and carbohydrate food(s).
- Walk, while eating and drinking, for at least a mile.

Recovery

- Within the first 30 minutes after finishing, eat a snack of about 200–400 calories. Try to have a 4:1 ratio of carbohydrates to protein. The Endurox R4 sports drink has this ratio and has been shown to speed recovery.
- If possible, immerse your legs for 10–20 minutes in a cool bath within 3 hours after the finish.

- Later in the day, walk for 30 to 60 minutes.
- Eat carbohydrate snacks continuously the rest of the day.
- Drink at least four to six ounces of water or electrolyte fluids every hour.
- The next day, walk for 30 to 60 minutes.
- Two days after the marathon, run and walk for 30 to 45 minutes.
- On the days following, continue to alternate: walk for between 30 and 60 minutes and run/walk for between 30 and 45 minutes.
- Wait at least a week before you schedule your next race or vow never to do another marathon.

"The marathon is a race for champions. It is not only about physical endurance but also mental and emotional endurance and strength. I used to think I was more of a 'solo' runner but since I have been training with 'my' Galloway running group I have learned that I gain endurance and strength from the group. . . .

Marathoning for me is not only about putting one foot in front of the other for 26 miles, it is about sharing stories with others I most likely would not have met had we not had the common goal of staying upright and feeling good for 26.2 miles. We each come to the marathon with our own goals, desires, and dreams and find along the way others who have something to teach us."

—Margot Springfield

15 RECOVERY AND BEYOND

Even if you've run twice as far as you've ever raced before in your life, you can be back to your normal running routine very quickly by following a few simple steps, before and after the race. By mentally and physically preparing for the morning after, you can reduce the negatives, while emotionally riding the wave of positive momentum from even the toughest of races.

The post-race letdown

Even with the best preparation, however, there will be a natural motivational lull. When they have spent months working toward a specific event and have reached the finish line of a significant physical test, even the most focused athletes experience a psychological letdown. The challenge has motivated you to be regular with your exercise, to keep pushing your endurance limits on long runs, and to reach down deep for motivation and the strength to go on. Like any significant accomplishment, the day of achievement marks an emotional peak and is invariably followed by a downturn. As soon as you grasp the reality that the "accomplishment doldrums" will occur,

you can prepare for them and desensitize yourself. Talk yourself through this: "It's natural, after six months of preparation for the big day, to miss the focus, the commitment, and the reinforcement of others who supported me in my mission." But you can also tell yourself with honesty that in a few days you can be shrugging off the blues as you strike out in a new direction.

Another mission

So, let's get another mission started, *now*! Write the date of your next project on a calendar or in a journal. It's best to shift gears and select a different type of mission: a scenic trail run, a weekend trip to a big festival event, a group run with friends you haven't seen for a while, and so on. If you've trained in a group, schedule an easy group run three to four weeks after the race, and you'll look forward to the reunion. It's okay to shift missions in midstream, but be sure to have a specific event always written on the calendar. If you wait until after your first "mission day" to choose another goal, your letdown will be more severe.

The body follows your mental mission

The more you embrace your new mission in advance, the quicker you'll lose the aches and pains of the big race. Instead of wallowing in your misery, tell yourself that your muscles have achieved their "good tiredness" by overcoming a great challenge—and you're still glowing from it. The positive mental momentum of your accomplishment will pull you through the few days immediately after when you may (or may not) feel that the legs don't want to run a step. Read this section several times before your event, mentally rehearsing each of the elements.

Whatever you do, don't stop moving

Begin your recovery program at the finish line. Even if you don't want to, keep walking. Grab two cups of water, drink, and keep walking. Get two more cups and pour them on your legs and two more on your head if you feel hot. Walk to the food area, pick up your carbohydrate snacks of choice (foods that have a 4:1 ratio of carbohydrates to protein are best), and eat, while you continue drinking water or an electrolyte beverage. Keep walking for a mile or so —your legs will recover faster because the walking pumps new blood in there, pushing the waste products out.

Throughout the afternoon

If possible, soak the legs in a cool tub of water for 15 minutes. (Cool faucet tap water is OK.) Drink water, electrolyte beverages, or citrus juice and eat some low-fat protein with other carbohydrates. You've earned your food rewards, and you'll reload most effectively when you've eaten a good small meal within 30 minutes of the finish. You don't have to be a pig; just keep snacking all afternoon and evening. For the next few days, you may want to increase your consumption of vitamin C to speed up the healing of microtears in your muscles and tendons.

The next day

On the following day, walk for 30 to 60 minutes or more. The pace can be as slow as you wish, just keep moving. If you have soreness, the walking will work it out quicker than sitting on a couch will.

Two days after

Begin running again, but start by walking for five to 10 minutes. Then, insert a 1-minute run break every 3 to 5 minutes. Stay out there for 30 to 60 minutes, adjusting the walking and running so that you feel comfortable and are not straining. The return to short segments of gentle running will speed up the recovery of race-weary muscles even more.

The next two weeks

Continue to alternate running days with walking days over the next two weeks. Walk for 30 to 60 minutes one day and follow that with a day of walk-running for 30 to 60 minutes. Gradually increase the running portions. Four days after the race, for example, you could try walking for 3 minutes and jogging for 2 or 3 minutes. Two days later, you may be back to running for 3 minutes and walking for 1 minute. Don't push yourself and you'll recover faster.

Don't race yet

Take one week off from racing and speed training for every six miles of the race you have just run. After a marathon, don't race for at least five weeks. You could schedule a short race three weeks after a half marathon. Even if you're feeling great, a 5K race run too soon after a marathon or half marathon can leave you more fatigued than you felt after your big race.

Resuming long runs

Run the weekend runs as they are listed on your training schedule, and run them slowly. A race longer than 15K up to 30K, such as a half marathon, will require a two- to three-week vacation from long runs. To run a 30K distance and beyond, the long run can be resumed three to four weeks after the race and every third week thereafter. As you resume long runs, be sure to pace them according to the Two-Minute Rule. Most runners will speed up their recovery if they run even more slowly on the long ones.

A growing number of marathoners are choosing to do their training runs in a different city's event each month. The self-proclaimed members of this fictitious Marathon-a-Month Club enjoy the travel with a mission and the different personality of each marathon. By doing these at least 2 minutes per mile slower than they could run on that day, and inserting all walk breaks, there is little risk of injury.

Your next marathon

If you've run a marathon and want to run another one in the near future, first, make sure that you have recovered. *(Consult the table on p. 103.)* Run the weekend runs as listed on the training schedule for the three weeks after the marathon. Once you've run 18 miles or more, you can maintain this level or increase your limit by running long every third weekend for at least 18 miles. Those who plan to run a marathon six to seven weeks later would have a 23- to 26-miler three weeks after the first marathon. If there are more than six to seven weeks between marathons, count back from marathon day. Three weeks before the second marathon, run 23 to 26 miles; three weeks before that, run 20 to 23, and so on.

Rely on the group

After every goal-oriented event, a few people are no longer motivated enough to continue running by themselves. The fun and the bonding that occurs in a training group that runs at a very comfortable pace for you will keep you running and can make running fun. When you have a choice, pick a group that runs at a pace that is slower than your usual pace. By running within your capacity, you'll be able to tell jokes and even remember some of the better ones. See p. 202 for a website that can connect you with training groups or, for those whose schedule or location prevents their joining a group, see p. 203 for training software.

That was great! What about the next one?

How soon after a marathon can I real-istically think of doing another one? It depends upon how close you ran to your potential, or maximum effort, in the most recent marathon. Here is a table giving you some guidelines:

If your pace was...	and your legs felt good in...	you can run the next one...
At least 2 minutes per mile slower	3–5 days	4 weeks later
At least one minute per mile slower	3–8 days	8 weeks later
At least one minute per mile slower	6–14 days	12+ weeks later
At least 30 seconds per mile slower	8–18 days	16+ weeks later
At least 30 seconds per mile slower	19–24 days	20+ weeks later
As fast as you could have run	NA	26+ weeks later

THE LITTLE THINGS THAT SPEED RECOVERY

- Start conservatively. Time-goal runners should start the race at a pace that is between 10 and 20 seconds slower than they feel that they could run on that day, and maintain that pace for at least the first 15 to 20 percent of the race (3 to 6 miles in a marathon). First-time marathoners should slow down by 1 to 2 minutes per mile. During the second half, you can choose to speed up or, for a faster recovery, to finish within your capacity. Even if it happens to be a hot, humid, bad day, you won't slow down as much at the end if you've started conservatively.

- Avoid alcohol and salt and limit caffeine during the 36 hours before the big day. In addi-tion, drink six to eight ounces of water or electrolyte beverage each hour until you hear sloshing in your stomach.

- Take *every* walk break, from the beginning, and pace yourself conservatively, accounting for heat, humidity, hills, and other factors.

- Don't over-stride at any time. Without knowing it, many runners are so exuberant in the beginning that they lengthen their stride too far, overextending the muscles. Then, more damage occurs from over-striding at the end of long runs and races—especially marathons. Rein in your stride as you go downhill. Studies continue to show that you'll run faster and recover faster when you keep your feet low to the ground, have a short stride, and stay light on your feet.

- During the second half of a run that will last 90 minutes or more, eat the Gel or Goo prod-ucts, pieces of energy bar, etc. all the way to the end. Be sure to drink water at the same time.

- Drink a few sips of water at every water stop, but no more than 20 oz. an hour.

"I ran the San Francisco Half Marathon, for no other reason than to make a trip to San Francisco, and run though a beautiful city on a lovely Sunday morning. I ran the first half last year, and figured I'd run the second half this year. I didn't train for this race in any special way. In fact, I didn't train for this race at all, other than to go out and run my daily runs, which often times don't exceed a couple of miles at a time. Since I didn't have any specific goals for this race, other than to get out there and run on Sunday morning, I decided to give the Run/Walk a try. I never thought of doing this myself, especially during a competitive race!

It worked out extremely well. In fact, it was the easiest 13.1 miles I've ever done. I started thinking that maybe I should have run the entire marathon, what the heck! In any case, toward the end of the race, other very kind and caring runners would encourage me during my walk breaks, saying 'It's not far now,' 'You can do it!' I turn to them and say 'Thanks, I'll see you in a few minutes!' And sure enough, others said, 'Hey, you were just walking,' or 'Not you again!' It was fun, and it definitely keeps your mind busy as you're awaiting the next walk break. As we were turning back into Golden Gate Park at the very end of the race, two guys passed me just as I was starting my run again, and I overheard them say, 'Hey, have you heard anything about this Run/Walk thing?' I turned around and said, 'It's fantastic.'"

–Sue Schlemmer

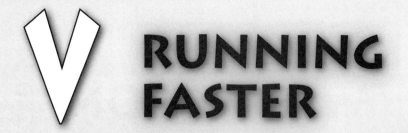

V RUNNING FASTER

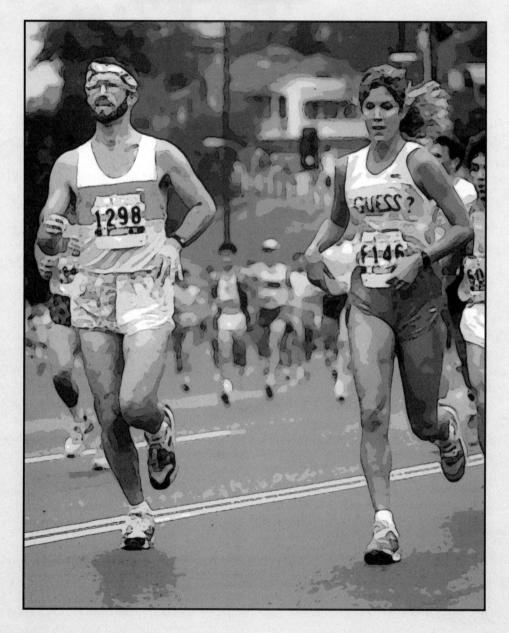

16 THE MARATHON IN REAL TIME

Training for a time goal increases injury risk by about 3 times.

Before you attempt a time-goal marathon, read this

There are many different marathon missions. Each can enrich your life in a different way and deliver about the same exhilaration as you experienced the first time.

Over the past twenty years, I must have compared notes with over fifty thousand veteran marathoners. A few continue to focus exclusively on running the fastest time they can run, every event. But almost every veteran, even those with more than a hundred completion medals, will put at the top of the rewards the unique feeling of satisfaction experienced every time the finish line is crossed.

Why run faster?

Good question! When the benefits are few and the challenges significant and many, you must answer this question before and throughout the program to maintain consistent motivation. Every person needs to dig down and come up with his or her own answer. I'll give you mine.

Most of the enduring and life-changing benefits from the marathon experience come only from finishing, but there are a few life-enhancing capabilities to be gained from testing yourself in a time-goal

marathon program. It's possible to get all of the benefit from this test, even if you don't do the marathon. It's also possible to have the good genes and or luck to run a fast time and receive none of the good internal engineering.

Finishing a marathon forces everyone to bring mind and body together and to reach for extra resources from the power of the human spirit. A time-goal marathon program goes one step farther than finishing, putting you on the edge of endurance and strength almost every week. In this process, you will invariably find weaknesses and setbacks. As you pull yourself out of a rut, you must question your resolve and your spirit, readjust, and come back stronger. Almost all the time-goal runners I've communicated with have been recharged by the challenge with a better understanding of who they are, as people. And many of those apply the lessons to other areas of life.

The time goal

Don't attempt a time goal until you have run at least one marathon. Even veteran runners will learn some very important lessons in their first marathon. Everyone can have a really good experience in that

FROM 2:38 TO 5:10 IN ONE YEAR . . . AND HAPPIER!

From my own experience, I can say that going from a 2:38 marathon to a 5:10 marathon was a definite improvement! A few years ago, I trained to run a marathon in less than 2:40. In spite of my 8- to 9-minutes-per-mile pace on daily runs, I believed that my forty-five-year-old legs could average 6 minutes per mile (all I needed to do was to add some regular speedplay to my program). A session of mile repeats every other week (building up to 13 and running each at 5:40) seemed to be doing the job. My longest run, three weeks before the race, was 29 miles (at 8:30 pace). Despite pushing the pace too fast in the middle of my target race, the Houston-Tenneco Marathon, I achieved my goal, with two seconds to spare!

Several months later, I was asked to help someone run his first marathon. He guessed that he could run a marathon in just over four hours, but stomach problems pushed us over the five-hour barrier for the first time in my marathon life. That 5:10 marathon was a much better experience than the faster one had been. I received the same satisfaction from finishing the slow one as I did from finishing the fast one. An even bigger benefit was revealed during the recovery.

Three days after my five-hour marathon, I was running smoothly, easily, and as fast as I wanted to run. There were no aches or pains and no lingering problems. Quickly and easily resuming my normal running program, I enjoyed the glow of satisfaction from having reestablished marathon endurance.

Four weeks after my 2:38 marathon, the pride of achieving my time goal had worn off, yet my running muscles were still stiff.

For several weeks, I continued to feel regular bouts of lingering tiredness. During those many weeks, I longed for the day when I'd feel smooth and fluid again.

I've articulated a pattern from analyzing many other slow and fast marathons that have been run by me and thousands of the folks with whom I work. The slower you go, particularly in the beginning, the faster you'll recover from the marathon. I believe very strongly that the satisfaction is identical whether you register a personal best, a personal worst, or anything in between. Finishing a marathon bestows great personal achievement and accomplishment. Period!

Certainly there is significant meaning in training for and realizing a time goal in the marathon. I recommend, however, that this be reserved for very few occasions (once every 12 to 24 months). When you enjoy a marathon and recover quickly afterward, you'll reinforce all of the positive behaviors and internal connections you've developed in the training. I believe that one should have at least three very slow and enjoyable marathons for every fast one—to keep the balance. I'm not denying that our egos are important sometimes and that some runners need to feed them with an occasional accomplishment. Don't give up the pursuit of a time goal if this is what you want. Just realize that focusing too exclusively on speed and time has led to burnout for many runners.

I want you to enjoy running for the rest of your life. So, take it easy!

first marathon if the start is slow and the pace kept comfortable throughout. A good first-time goal should be to finish a marathon about an hour slower than you could run the same distance if you were racing.

Predicted Goal Pace		
After 3–4 MMs	3% improvement	5% improvement
6 min/mi	5:48/mile	5:42/mile
7 min/mi	6:48/mile	6:39/mile
8 min/mi	7:46/mile	7:36/mile
9 min/mi	8:44/mile	8:33/mile
10 min/mi	9:42/mile	9:30/mile
11 min/mi	10:40/mile	10:27/mile
12 min/mi	11:38/mile	11:24/mile
13 min/mi	12:37/mile	12:21/mile
14 min/mi	13:35/mile	13:18/mile
15 min/mi	14:33/mile	14:15/mile
16 min/mi	15:31/mile	15:12/mile
17 min/mi	16:29/mile	16:09/mile
18 min/mi	17:27/mile	17:06/mile
19 min/mi	18:25/mile	18:03/mile
20 min/mi	19:23/mile	19:00/mile

*Weather influences finish times more than anything else. Every degree above 60°F will generate a slower finish time. The pace of long runs and the race itself should be slowed by 30 seconds per mile for every 5 degree increase above 60°F. The bottom line is that you must slow down long runs and races, from the beginning, on a day that is hotter than 60°F. Be prepared to adjust. Many of my Galloway runners bring a thermometer with them to make the adjustments as needed.

"Magic Mile" time trials (MM)

The *"Magic Mile" time trials (MM)* are reality checks on your goal. These should be done on the weeks noted on the schedule. These will tell us a realistic training pace, and what would be a hard pace for the marathon itself. With this information, you can make the decision about how hard to run. *(If you have any injuries you should not do the MM.)*

- Warm up for these with about 10 minutes of very easy running with liberal walk breaks.
- Do 4-6 accelerations as in the book—no sprinting.
- Run around a track if at all possible.
- Time yourself for 4 laps (1600 meters). Start the watch at the beginning, and keep it running until you cross the finish of the fourth lap.
- *On the first MM, don't run all-out: run at a pace that is slightly faster than your current pace.*
- Only one MM is done on each day it is assigned.
- On each successive MM (usually 3 weeks later), your mission is to beat the previous best time.
- Don't ever push so much that you hurt your feet, knees, etc.
- Jog slowly for the rest of the distance assigned on that day, taking as many walk breaks as you wish.

After you have run 3 of these (not at one time—on different weekends) you'll see progress and will run them hard enough so that you are huffing and puffing during the second half—and finish feeling like you couldn't go much further at that pace. Try walking for about 10–15 seconds at the mid-point (800 meters) during the MM. Some runners record a faster time when taking short breaks, and some go faster when running continuously. Do what works for you on the MM.

Running for time requires twice as much training

There are many drawbacks to setting a goal that is too challenging. If you enjoy the competition and the satisfaction of achieving a specific goal, then one or two marathons a year (at most) could be set aside for this purpose. The best reward for this hard work is the Boston Marathon. Qualifying for Boston is one of the greatest accomplishments in a runner's life. The experience of that special weekend, during which over a million people cheer you with unique intensity, will be something you'll remember the rest of your life.

Before committing yourself to a time-goal program, be sure to evaluate the ratio of risk to reward. To train so that you can finish a marathon requires very little interruption in your lifestyle. The extra training time required for a time goal can, however, take its toll on your family, career, and other areas of life. Training "to finish" takes about one-third to one-half the time required to train for most time-goal marathons. The extra mileage and speed training will also produce more aches, pains, doubts, discouraging messages, and, possibly, injuries.

The burnout factor There is a high burnout rate among time-goal marathoners. They often become so focused on the goal that they miss the joy of responding to an early morning run or the glow on a trail at sunset. If the satisfaction is derived solely from the clock at the finish, most of the joys of running slip by, underappreciated. One reason for the high rate of failure of marathoners to hit a specific goal is that they have no control over several of the primary reasons for slowing down in a marathon: temperature, humidity, the difficulty of the course, and the congestion of a crowded event.

Variations on the time goal

Time goals don't have to be limited to marathons run in the shortest possible time. Here are a few variations on the theme that have energized me and others. Don't stop with these ideas. Be creative and you'll look forward to every one.

- **Set up a reasonable time goal** — one that you know you can do. Tell your friends about it and see if they want to have a pool. The winner and the marathoner (you) get a free celebration dinner.

- **Beat a younger you** — a time you have run once before. Every ten years for 40 years, I ran the Atlanta Marathon, the event where I started my marathon career in 1963. My mission was to beat the time that I ran as an 18-year-old.

- **Set a maximum** — put a penalty on speed. This is a particularly good goal for those who find it hard to slow down. Punish yourself for finishing in less than a certain time. This has helped hundreds of runners to learn how to hold back and enjoy the company of those farther back in the pack.

Get a life!

If you include running fun, every week, and you're flexible about your goal, you can usually reach your time goal . . . and a life too. At least two of your long runs could be done in other marathons, gradually building up to the fast one (observe the Two-Minute Rule!). If the weather or your body doesn't cooperate on goal day, don't trash yourself. Slow down to training pace and you can usually recover fairly quickly — and race another marathon in 3–4 weeks.

The slow marathon

I've run over 90 marathons the recreational way. By running more slowly than I could run, from the beginning, the marathon becomes enjoyable. When I ran the Boston Marathon with my father in 1996, I had already run Boston four times previously. Because I was going along comfortably, I enjoyed the course and was surprised to recognize very little of it. Each of the other efforts had been fiercely competitive. I hardly noticed anything but the clock, my competitors, and how I felt. It was so much better in 1996, savoring the landmarks, the people, and the time with my Dad.

The more significantly you back off from the pace you could run, the better you'll feel during the marathon and the more likely it will be that you'll remember what went on. You'll expand the number of possible running companions and enrich the time you are spending covering those 26 miles.

Use this evolving "story line" as you move from marathon to marathon.

Alternatives to a time goal

Help a charity A growing number of runners find it fulfilling to raise money for a charity that means something to them. Many charities have programs that allow donors to deduct the contributions from their taxes while the runner earns a free trip to a great marathon. I support the Marathon to Fight Breast Cancer in Jacksonville, FL—a great event (donation by entry fee).

Run with a relative I've heard it said numerous times that there's no better way to see relatives in a positive light than to train with that person and then run a marathon together. The bonding is impossible to describe. When you live in different cities, the phone contact throughout the training keeps you in touch and your relationship alive.

Mentor someone who really needs it At every marathon expo, I talk with folks who are reunited by training for and running a marathon together. Maybe you want to reconnect with a college roommate who is going through a divorce or introduce a high school best friend to your marathon training buddies. It could be a former mentor of yours who has lost fitness and focus and is looking for both. Marathon training helps people restart their lives (or reconnect) in a positive way.

Run in 50 states After running five to ten marathons, some new marathoners like the challenge and the travel. So they set out on a five- to ten-year goal to run a marathon in every state. This has been extended to all continents, Canadian provinces, and so on. Whatever makes sense to you is an appropriate mission!

Revisit a special place It could be the town where you or your father grew up, went to college, started your career—whatever is interesting to you.

A scavenger hunt If someone in your group knows the course, you can set up a scavenger hunt. Buy souvenirs from certain parts of town on the course, wear pieces of clothing from distinctive stores, or take a "throwaway" camera and get pictures of yourself with landmarks on the course for proof. Your imagination is your only limit.

Sightseeing, with a list Carry a little notepad and pen in your fanny pack and note the historical and scenic points on the course. Try to find something about each area that most people would overlook. This gives you a creative task during walk breaks. Compare notes with friends at your victory celebration afterward.

QUESTIONS

"I've tried to run a marathon slowly, and I became more sore than I was after a fast one."

If you're getting sore or feeling the need to expend more effort when going slowly, then you're running inefficiently. By shortening your stride and keeping the feet low to the ground, you waste very little effort. In this very efficient running mode, your main running muscles are mostly resting.

I've talked to several fast runners who seem to be running correctly, yet still became sore after a marathon. After a few more questions, I learned, however, that they went into the marathon with the longest run of their training being only 19, 16, or, in one case, 6 miles. Whenever you ask your body to go that much further than it has gone in the recent past, you can predict that there'll be some retribution from your muscles afterward.

To reduce the chance of soreness, take walk breaks early and often.

"Why should I waste a marathon by running slowly? How can you run a slow marathon? You have to train for six months and I want to make the most of this challenge."

I understand. For my first 60 marathons, I was a competitor. When the gun fired, the force of my being was directed at reaching the finish line as I would in any race: with nothing left. I ran some fast times (*e.g.*, a 2:16) but I did not enjoy these experiences. When I placed well, such as a win at Honolulu and fifth- and seventh-place finishes at Boston, the afterglow was compromised by weeks of soreness, tiredness, blisters, and wounded ego (I always felt, even when I ran well, that I could have run faster).

17 TO RUN FASTER, YOU MUST TRAIN FASTER

You can't run all of your runs slowly if you want to run fast in the marathon. But you can't go too fast either. By running the speed play too fast, for example, you will prepare your muscles to go out too fast in the marathon and pay dearly for that later. The best type of speed simulates the marathon experience. This will encourage the particular adaptations of endurance and speed that will be necessary if you are to go faster on race day.

Strength and coordination are developed simultaneously with the other improvements generated by speed sessions.

The cardiovascular system adapts:

- The heart pumps more blood into the exercising muscles.
- Waste products are withdrawn more quickly from those muscles.

Your oxygen-processing system becomes more efficient:

- Oxygen is absorbed more efficiently from the air.
- Oxygen is delivered to the muscles to allow you to burn fat longer.

Adaptations also occur inside the muscles:

- Fat burning makes you more efficient.

- You become more efficient when burning glycogen.
- Individual muscle cells work at a higher capacity for a longer period and muscle cells learn to work together, in systems; for more information on the changes in muscles, see *Galloway's Book on Running,* pp. 38–43.

You develop the mental strength to go further:

- You develop instant and continuous feedback between the mind and the body.
- You learn how to dig deeper and push through doubt.
- You learn the difference between real problems and the stressed messages of your left brain.

The danger in speed

But every time you run fast, you increase the chance of injury, you stress and fatigue the main running muscles, and you increase the chance that you'll not recover before the marathon itself. To do your best in the marathon, all of your components should be ready for top performance, working together, and trained to make further adaptations under stress. The stress of speed play is necessary if you are to run faster, but you need to monitor fatigue to avoid injury or over-training.

Recovery, recovery, recovery

The main theme of a time-goal program is recovery. If you build enough rest into your program before you need it, your body will be continuously recovering, rebuilding, and adapting for the performance demands of your goal. By preventing extra fatigue and taking extra rest at even the first hint of slower recovery, you can maintain a steady performance increase without being forced to take a week or more off because of injury or over-training.

Make sure that you take:

- Enough days off from running each week
- Long runs that are slow enough—with walk breaks (at least 2 minutes per mile slower than realistic marathon pace)
- Walks during the rest interval between mile repeats
- The beginning of every run very slowly (at least 3 minutes per mile slower than you could run the distance you plan to run). You can speed up later in the run if everything is okay; *just start very slowly.*
- Time to make sure that you are recovered enough from the weekend sessions before you do any race-pace running *(see "Marathon Rehearsal," p. 128)*, accelerations *(see pp. 115–116 and 129)*, etc. during the maintenance runs on weekdays.

Monitoring stress

Keep a log book Record your pulse rate before you get out of bed each morning. Do this even before you've had a chance to think about anything stressful, such as getting up, work, and so on.

Why? When your exercising muscles are over-fatigued, they don't have the resilience to help move the blood through the system in the smoothest way. The heart must work harder and registers this with a higher heart rate.

When to take a day off? After several weeks of listing your heart rate, you'll be able to tell what your baseline levels are. When you see a 5 percent increase over your baseline, you should take an easy day. When the heart rate is 10 percent above baseline, just take the day off from running.

Remember that heart rate is affected not only by stress, but also by elation and other emotions and thoughts. Try not to think about anything before taking your pulse.

Adding mileage

By adding mileage to your program, you'll improve your overall conditioning and improve the chance that you can achieve your time goal. But higher mileage dramatically increases the risk of injury. By a wide margin it is the leading cause of injury. But, there are some ways to increase total mileage and reduce the chance of injury:

- Increase the mileage very gradually.
- Add a short additional run to a running day.
- Start and finish your running days with a mile of very slow running (at least 3 minutes per mile slower than your current 5K pace).
- Be aware of all the early warning signs of injury or over-fatigue and back off at the first indication of trouble.

How many days a week?

Almost every marathoner, including most of those training for the Olympic Trials could benefit from two days off from running per week. Age will determine, and ultimately dictate, how many more days off you will need. If you experience an increase in fatigue, aches, or feel tired on most runs, consider extra days off from running:

- Those in their thirties can get by with two days off per week.

- If you are in your forties, you had better take three days off from running per week.

- If you're over fifty, it's best to run only every other day.

- If you've been running six or seven days a week, I would suggest that you start by cutting back by one day per week. As the long runs reach 15 miles and beyond, cut one more day out of the schedule. You can actually increase your mileage on running days by adding another run (if the recovery is proceeding well). Other types of exercise can be done on non-running days, but take it very easy the day before you do your long run, races, and speed play.

A fastest marathon at age 62

As he approached the age of 60, Dr. George Sheehan's marathon times slowed down. For years, he had been running 5 miles a day, six days a week. Admitting that his competitive days appeared to be over, the cardiologist cut back to three days a week, while increasing his daily mileage to 10 miles. In other words, his mileage held steady at 30 miles per week, but he gained three extra rest days.

After about three years of this schedule, at the age of 62, George ran the fastest marathon of his life: 3:01. He had gained more training effect from one 10-miler than he ever had from two successive 5-milers. Even more significant was the improved recovery attained because he was taking a day off between runs.

Older runners

Because it is possible to continue to improve your times at any age, many runners over the age of 45 are so elated when they run personal records or turn in fast age-group performances that they forget that they're over the hill. The exuberance of achievement will push runners at any age into over-fatigue before they know it; the older the runner, the longer he or she has to pay for the excessive training.

Unfortunately, there are few early warning signs of over-training in a marathon program. Most of those who get into trouble are increasing their endurance gradually enough, but they just don't have adequate recovery time built into their programs. The progressive buildup pushes the muscles beyond their limits so gradually that the effects are usually masked by internally produced stress hormones. But, once the resource reserve has been used up, older runners must endure a long recovery period.

To avoid fatigue, set limits on:

- the days of running per week
- the miles run per week
- the number of races run
- the number of speed sessions
- very long long runs

If you're over 35

When you are past the age of 35, fatigue sets in more quickly but is usually masked by stress hormones. It's easier to push yourself into over-training without seeing any warning signs. Then, the worse the over-training, the longer the recovery: it takes 2–3 times as long for people over 40 to recover from fatigue as it does for those younger than 30 and between five and six times longer to recover from severe fatigue.

To reduce the chance of injury when you are over the age of 35, you should:

- Add an extra day off (you will still need to run a minimum of three days per week).
- Limit the long runs to a pace of 3 minutes per mile slower than you could run that day.
- Add walk breaks to long runs, from the beginning.
- In speed sessions walk for at least 2 to 3 minutes during the rest interval.
- Monitor your resting heart rate carefully.

Long runs can improve your speed

By increasing beyond 26 miles, you'll build reserve endurance that will boost your performance in several ways:

- You'll push your fatigue "wall" past 26 miles.
- You'll have the strength and stamina to maintain a hard pace during the last 3 to 6 miles, when most competitive folks slow down.
- With reserve endurance, you can often get away with a few small pacing mistakes.

- Those who increase their longest run from 20 miles to 26 miles show a range of improvement of 10 to 20 minutes.
- Those who increase their longest run from 26 miles to 29 miles show a range of improvement of 5 to 13 minutes.

Go *slow* in the long runs

You get the same benefit from a long slow run as you do from a long fast one and you'll recover faster from the slow run. If you go further than 20 miles in the long run, you will improve your marathon stamina dramatically but you must run slowly. Remember that running more slowly will help you to recover faster and keep the legs ready to do speed sessions on the following weekend.

> By pacing these long runs at least 2 minutes per mile slower than predicted by the "magic mile," and by taking the appropriate walk breaks, you'll get the job done!

Liberal walk breaks will also speed recovery from long runs. Those 1-minute walks must be taken early and often to give your legs the relief needed. Also, make sure that the maintenance runs during the week are done slowly enough. Sometimes a slight bit of fatigue will appear on the second or third day after a long run or a speed session. Take it very easy if that happens.

Acceleration gliders

To improve running form and efficiency, accelerations can help you greatly. When your form improves, your speed will naturally increase as well. Acceleration is a technique that improves your fast running technique while allowing you to glide or coast for distances of between 20 and 60 meters, resting the major running muscles so that they will perform better later. Acceleration gliders will warm up the legs before speed sessions, hills, or races. And, by focusing on these gliders, you teach yourself efficient marathon running form.

How to do acceleration gliders

1. To get momentum going, it helps to have a slight downhill. Use the last 20 to 30 meters of the downhill to get right into gliding at an increased pace, being sure to keep the legs and body relaxed throughout, but particularly at the beginning.

2. If no downhill is available, jog slowly for 15 steps, jog faster for 15 steps, then gradually accelerate by shortening your stride length and gradually increasing the turnover of your feet and legs for 15–20 steps. (Turnover is simply the number of steps you take per minute.)

3. When you feel comfortable at the faster rhythm, maintain a short stride, touch lightly, and let the ankle move you forward with little effort.

4. You're touching quickly, so just glide, keeping the feet low to the ground and using very little effort, gradually slowing down.

5. Continue gliding for between 20 and 60 meters.

6. Rest by jogging between accelerations. You may also take walk breaks as needed.

Your acceleration glider program

- Work on marathon form as described on pp. 23–27.
- Warm up before each session with 1 to 2 miles of easy running (with walk breaks if you wish).
- Keep the legs relaxed throughout the warm-up, the gliders themselves, and afterward.
- Ease into the gliders, using downhills as the accelerations. If you don't have a downhill available, accelerate by shortening the stride, picking up the turnover rate of the legs, and then let the ankles move you forward.
- Start with 3 to 5 gliders and increase by 1 or 2 each session to a maximum of 8.
- It's important to do this drill at least once a week to maintain form improvements.
- You can use these as a warm-up before hills, speed sessions, or races. You may also do them during your recovery and maintenance runs each week.

"My goal was to run the Ocean State Marathon under 4:30 and I finished in 4:27. When I was taking a walk break, a man next to me said 'C'mon, keep going.' I told him what I was doing and he didn't seem to understand. The best part was when I passed him later in the race."

—Stephanie Elterich
New York City

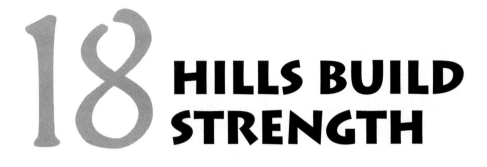

18 HILLS BUILD STRENGTH

Hill training provides a gentle and effective transition between very slow running and the faster speed play needed by veteran marathoners for faster performance. If you're just starting to run, you shouldn't jump into hill play. But those who've been running regularly for six months or more can benefit from the increase in strength that only hill training can give. You don't need to have a time goal to benefit from play on the hills.

Hills for muscle power

Hills provide resistance to the main running muscle groups, primarily the calf muscles. The regular but gentle uphill stress encourages these muscles to develop strength in the act of running.

When runners of all ability levels run hill sessions regularly, they develop the lower leg strength to support body weight farther forward on their feet. As the foot rolls forward in the running motion, better support will allow the ankle to be loaded like a strong spring. The result is a continued, energetic lift-off of the foot as the ankle releases its mechanical energy, mile after mile. Due to the incredible efficiency of the ankle, more work is done with less energy expended by the muscles. Such conservation of muscle resources allows one to run further or faster, or a combination of both. Hill training also strengthens a set of muscles that are used as back-ups for the main running muscles and helps the cardiovascular system adapt to faster running without going into oxygen debt.

If you're doing hill training for the first time, be conservative. It's too easy to run too fast in the first few sessions without realizing it. *Don't push the effort!* Run at a comfortable, slow pace on each incline during the first few hill sessions. The grade of the hill will be enough of a challenge to bestow a training effect. After three hill play sessions, you may run the hills a little faster.

What about weight training for runners?

Weight training, in contrast, builds static strength in only one range of motion at a time. Weight work can strengthen some leg muscle groups more than others (and knock your running motion off balance), so it is not recommended for runners.

Hill training rules

- Never run all out!
- Never go to the point that you're not recovering between hills.

- Don't run so hard that you feel pain, cramping, or extreme exertion in any of the muscles or tendons in the back of your legs. If this happens, slow down immediately and shorten your stride. (The lengthening of the running stride beyond its efficient range can cause extra fatigue, if not injury, and require a long recovery.)

- No racing against your running companions during hill sessions! In any group, the runners' legs may be in varying stages of conditioning and may not be as warmed up as they should be. Injuries occur when you try to stay with someone who is feeling good and is in better condition than you are.

Hill training basics

- Take a very slow 1- to 2-mile warm-up and warm-down.

- Pick a hill according to running experience: beginners, 50 steps; advanced beginners, 100 steps; runners, 200 steps; competitors, 300 steps.

- The grade of the hill should be very gentle.

- Run up; walk down.

- Run with a smooth, continuous effort over the top of the hill.

- Never sprint or run all out. Just maintain an increased turnover rate until you're over the top.

- Start with two or three hills, and increase by one or two hills per week until you can run between eight and ten hills.

- Don't feel that you have to increase the number each session. Back off if you are tired or sore.

Make sure that you keep your stride length short to maintain turnover without tension in leg muscles. Avoid overexertion, and avoid extending your lower leg too far in front of you.

As in the other elements of training, it's important for hill sessions to be done regularly if they are to produce the adaptations desired from the legs and muscles and to improve your overall running efficiency. Hills will prepare the running muscles for a higher level of performance, so the more weekly sessions of hill running that you do, the more you will benefit from the added strength and running efficiency when you shift to speed play. When speed sessions begin, hill training is terminated.

Levels of running experience

- **Beginners**, who've been running for less than three months and have never done any kind of speed play

- **Advanced beginners**, who've been running for more than three months but have never done speed play

- **Runners**, who've been running for more than six months and have done some speed play

- **Competitors**, who've been running for years and have done regular periods of speed play

The grade of a hill is measured as a percentage, horizontal being 0 percent and perpendicular being 100 percent.

Beginners should choose hills with only a very slight grade, 1 to 2 percent. More experienced runners should play on hills with a 3 to 4 percent grade. Competition-level runners can choose hills with a 5 to 6 percent grade.

Scheduling

Run hills on weekends when you are not taking a long run and before marathon speed play begins. Or run hill repeats on a short day during the week.

Warm-up and warm-down for hills

A good walk of five minutes gets the blood flowing and the tendons and muscles warmed up. Start running very slowly, and jog for at least half a mile before doing any hills. Then do 4 acceleration gliders. The warm-down should reverse the warm-up.

Hill form

- Your goal is to develop a running form that is easier, lighter on the feet, and requires less effort. With repetition, the resistance provided by the hill will strengthen the lower legs. Bouncing, high push-offs, and long strides are counterproductive to marathon hill form. On the flat, many runners aren't aware of the imperfections in their form. But the extra effort required going up will aggravate any flaws. By increasing leg and foot turnover, you can often run faster while you run more smoothly.

- **Relax.** Don't contract the muscles or strain to keep the right alignment.

- **Stay upright.** Head over shoulders, over hips, and all three are lined up over the feet as they assume the weight of your body. Your alignment should be perpendicular to the horizontal and not to the incline of the hill. In this way, you're most efficiently distributing the weight of your body as it interacts with gravity.

- **Shorten your stride.** Keep shortening the stride until you feel a slight relaxing of the hamstring muscles at the back of the thigh. If your stride is too short, the choppy steps and loss of fluid motion will make you feel as if you are slowing down. Too long a stride causes tightness in the hamstrings and/or in the quadriceps muscles and significantly more effort is required for only a small increase in speed.

- **Keep your feet low.** The less you have to lift your feet, the more effort you'll conserve.

- **Quick turnover** To improve speed and strength, gradually increase the cadence or turnover of your legs and feet.

- **As the hill gets tougher,** keep reducing your stride length while trying to maintain or increase the turnover of your legs and feet. Remember, stay light on your feet and keep those feet low to the ground.

Beginner hill play

Grade: 1 to 2 percent; so easy that you barely feel the incline

Distance of hill segment: 50 to 60 meters; about half a city block

Pace: About the same as your easy running on flat land; no huffing or puffing

Recovery: Walk slowly down the hill and continue walking at the bottom for as long as needed.

Number of hills: Two or three hills on the first session, with an additional hill each week until you reach a comfortable number; a maximum of between eight and ten hills

Advanced beginner hill play

Grade: 1 to 2 percent; so easy that you barely feel the incline

Distance of hill segment: 100 meters

Pace: A little faster than your easy running on the flat, but no sprinting

Recovery: Walk slowly down the hill and continue walking for 3 to 5 minutes at the bottom and more if needed.

Number of hills: Start with two or three hills and build to between eight and ten hills.

Runner hill play

Grade: 3 to 4 percent; easy for the runner but steeper than hills for beginners

Distance of hill segment: 200 meters

Pace: No faster than that of a 10K race and usually slower

Recovery: Walk slowly down the hill and continue walking for 3 to 5 minutes at the bottom.

Number of hills: Start with between two and four hills and build to between eight and ten hills.

Competitor hill play

Grade: 5 to 6 percent; pick a grade that will allow you to maintain a steady speed and turnover all the way up the hill and over the top; if that means a flatter grade, that's fine.

Distance of hill segment: 300 meters

Pace: About that of a 5K race, adjusted to maintain smoothness, relaxed leg muscles, and turnover

Recovery: Jog and walk down the hill and continue walking for 2 to 3 minutes at the bottom.

Number of hills: Start with three to four hills and build to between eight and ten hills.

LONGER HILLS FOR SPEED DEMONS

- Run longer hills.
- Run the hills with no strong push off, running smoothly, but hard.
- Maintain a quick, smooth cadence so as to run up the hill with more strength.
- If you feel that the stride length is a bit short, maintain a stride that feels normal.

QUESTIONS

"Won't these longer hills keep me tired?"

Not if you run them with the short stride described above. Through practice, you'd be amazed how fast you can turn your legs over when going uphill. By not overextending the hamstring or calf muscles, your legs feel reasonably fresh, even at the end of the session.

"How do I speed up the turnover?"

Don't expect it to happen all at once. First, ensure that the hamstrings are loose and ready to respond to a quick turnover. The difference between the shortened stride and a stride that feels fully extended may be only an inch or so. You need only a slight shortening of the stride to relax the main running muscles. Relaxed muscles are more resilient, can respond quicker, and return to do it again quicker. This means quicker turnover. Stay low to the ground and touch lightly.

Short uphill stride rules

I ran my fastest marathon at the age of 35. The 1980 Houston-Tenneco course had several significant rolling sections, and this worried me. I had strained my hamstring eight weeks before the race and had to refrain from running fast. As the marathon date neared, I discovered that the only speed sessions I could do were hill repeats with a shortened stride. Although the injury was not completely healed, I picked up the turnover and jokingly told myself that I was the fastest "short strider" in the United States!

The hill's resistance gave me the quality of speed play needed to run a high-performance marathon. The shorter stride released the tension on the hamstring and allowed it to continue healing. Not only did I recover while doing quality work, I passed about two dozen competitors while going up hills in the race itself. They were huffing and puffing and I was zooming by at my normal respiration rate. I ran a strong race right to the finish in a lifetime best of 2:16.

"The three of us finished the hilly race in respectable times and most importantly with smiles on our faces. I never thought I could finish one marathon, let alone two marathons in five weeks' time! The 'power of the group' and learning the Galloway method of running got me there!"

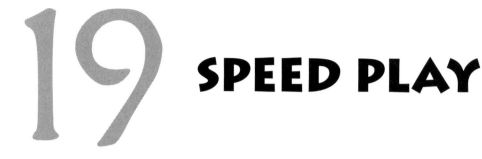

19 SPEED PLAY

Let me introduce you to a new type of speed session, one that offers the invigoration of going fast and the satisfaction of knowing you're getting better. You'll be able to joke with friends or yourself throughout the session and play games to keep the experience interesting.

Starting now, we have abolished the old, archaic speed work and replaced it with clean, upbeat, uplifting speed play. You're going to like it so much that you'll finish each session wanting to do more. And because you don't do more than the work assigned, you'll look forward to the next session.

It's got to be fun!

Set up your speed session in an interesting area. You can also change the venue if variety helps make it more interesting. Bring music, a clock (if possible), and banners that are funny, inspirational, or instill pride. Some runners bring along a few posters with uplifting graphics.

Many runners like to read something before the speed session. Whether it is humorous, entertaining, or informative, any reading will offer the chance that the left brain will be preoccupied so that it won't bother you with negative messages and excuses.

- Require each member to bring to each session (1) a joke, (2) a controversial viewpoint, and (3) some spicy news.
- Set up games in which runners of all abilities can run the same repetition, with the winner being the one closer to his or her assigned pace.
- Alternate the jokes, etc. so that there is a continuous flow of entertainment, at least during rest intervals.
- Use the walking between repetitions for other fun activities.

Speed play with a group

Running with others will improve morale, increase and maintain motivation, and make the session more fun. You can start together, but don't run at the pace of someone who is faster than you are. When in doubt, take more rest between repetitions, even if others in the group do not.

Numbers Groups are organized according to marathon time goals so that there are at least three to five runners in each group, to a maximum of about fifteen; the ideal size is eight to ten.

Timing Ideally, a digital display clock is available and each runner can see his or her time for each lap. Next best is to have a volunteer reading out the time for each lap. This job can rotate among the runners who are walking between mile repeats. In each case, the continuous time is read out. Each runner could track his or her pace by noting the time at the start of each mile and subtracting it from the total time at the finish. *Example:* A runner waited for the clock to click over to exactly 30 minutes as she started her fourth mile repeat. She finished in 40:40, doing the mile in exactly 10:30 (for an 11-minute-per-mile time-goal pace in the marathon).

Starting Each group starts together, with some runners straggling throughout each mile. Within each group there will usually be three to five different pace goals represented, so individuals need to be very aware of their own goal pace from the beginning of each mile.

Leadership Each pace group should have a group leader who helps to infuse fun, holds back those who are going out too fast, and encourages more walking between repeats for those who aren't resting enough.

Picking your goal

The most important part of the speed development process is the very first step: picking a goal that is realistic for you. "Magic Mile" (MM) Time Trials give you a reality check before your goal race.

- Try to run every one of the MMs on the schedule.
- Adjust pace on each lap so that you run a little faster during the last 2 laps.
- *Hint:* Hold yourself back on the first lap.
- Most runners will improve the MM on most attempts if training is done and rest days are taken.

- If you are not making progress, look for reasons and take action.
- The fastest time run during the last few MMs will predict a very hard race pace.
- You can then adjust your pace due to temperature and effort level desired.

It's okay if your goal is slower than you are currently capable of running. This strategy has led to many personal records. By setting yourself up for a performance that has some challenge but is realistic, you will take pressure off, stay in your right brain longer, and often run at a much higher level.

> If your goal is too far ahead of your ability, you set yourself up for disappointment and fatigue. By overestimating your capacity, you'll force yourself to run the speed sessions too fast and won't recover between speed days and long runs.

You'll be fine-tuning your racing form and technique after you've run two or three MMs. If the courses were hilly or the weather conditions were adverse, estimate the time you honestly believe you could run under better conditions. The prediction formulas give equivalent performances for many race distances, including the marathon, based upon ideal conditions and training.

If your MM performances don't predict the time you'd like, swallow your pride and select a less ambitious time goal. Slow down the pace of the mile repeats and your early pace in the marathon. *Always be conservative in choosing your goal.* If the MM performances predict a 4:30 marathon, shoot for 4:40 or 4:45. It's always better to finish the marathon knowing that you could have run faster: you've already started the momentum and have the motivation to do it.

Marathon speed work is different

Running faster in the marathon requires that you develop a special type of **speed/endurance.** The actual pace of the speed segments is only slightly faster than marathon goal pace. You're developing the capacity to maintain a moderate pace over a long distance. Compared with speed sessions for shorter distance racing, those for the marathon emphasize building endurance by longer repetitions (usually mile repeats) or by an increased number of repetitions, up to 14 of the mile repeats; faster marathons require more repetitions.

As you develop the capacity to run mile after mile in the time you need, you gain a sense of pace. It's actually detrimental to run the mile repeats faster than your schedule prescribes, which is 30 seconds faster than goal pace. If you exceed this speed limit, even in the beginning of the speed session, it becomes difficult for your internal pace clock to acquire the judgment needed in the marathon itself. A fast start will either leave you struggling at the end of the session or produce tired muscles that require a long recovery.

Recovery, recovery, recovery!

We mentioned it before, but the need for recovery cannot be overemphasized. Because the long runs and the speed sessions are fatiguing, everything possible should be done to speed up your recovery.

- Adhere strictly to the pace of the speed repetitions to avoid going too fast.
- Take a 5-minute walk between each mile repeat.
- Schedule enough easy days (and easy running) between the weekend sessions.

- Use the run-walk-run strategy you plan to use in your race, but take a walk break that is half the amount you plan to use during the race itself.

Where?

A track is not necessary. Accurately measured road segments, a park, well-packed trails, or other safe venues are just as good. Wherever you run, make sure that the mile is accurately measured. During the first few sessions, a track can help by giving regular timed feedback, usually every quarter mile. This helps to set your internal pace clock more quickly. It's more fun to listen to music as you make the loops of the oval. When choosing a road segment, avoid downhills that are too steep or give you too much advantage. Likewise, avoid uphills that are too steep and will force you either to slow down or to overwork to maintain the pace.

How often?

To encourage the useful adaptations and improvements in form, rhythm, etc., speed sessions must be done regularly, that is, on the designated weekends when you are not doing a long run, starting about 16 weeks before the marathon. By adding other innovations to your program, such as race rehearsal pace runs during the week, you'll maintain and extend the faster running form and performance benefits gained from speed sessions in all of your runs.

Warm-up

Whatever speed play format you choose, get the blood flowing through the muscles with a gentle warm-up. This introduction to exercise allows the tendons, ligaments, and muscles to warm up together and begin working as a team. A good warm-up will decrease the chance of injury and increase the intuitive cooperation of components within the muscles.

- Walk for 5 to 10 minutes.
- Jog *very* slowly for 5 minutes.
- Jog for another 5 minutes at a comfortable pace.
- Do 4 acceleration gliders.
- Walk for 2–3 minutes.

On days when the muscles are feeling tight some runners require one extra mile of extra easy walking and running to warm up. As we age, we need more slow warm-up distance at the beginning of every run. When it comes to the warm-up, slower is always better.

Stretching

If you want to stretch before running, be careful. Stretching the wrong way before running may increase your chance of injury. It's easy to over-stretch a muscle that hasn't been used much and thus leave the muscles tighter than they were before and more susceptible to injury. Don't make the mistake of trying to loosen up a tight muscle by stretching the heck out of it. Tight muscles tell you that you need to ease off until they feel loose.

A slow walk followed by very slow running and walking for 10 to 15 minutes will allow the muscles to relax and warm up better than stretching. For more information on stretching and for specific, useful stretches, see *Galloway's Book on Running*.

Mile repeats

The most popular form of marathon speed play is interval training, a technique that has been used by world-class athletes for many,

many years. Measured segments (repetitions) are run at a pace that is slightly faster than marathon goal pace and are followed by a rest interval. This process is repeated many times. Shorter-distance goal races, such as the 5K and 10K, use short repetitions of between 400 and 800 meters. Longer repetitions, such as mile repeats, have been overwhelmingly the most successful distance used in the Galloway program. 800-meter repetitions can be useful for the marathon, but the mile distance helps to mold together the components of marathon form and exertion in one exercise.

BENEFITS OF MILE REPEATS

- They force your legs and feet to find more efficient ways of running, by, for example, eliminating or significantly reducing extraneous motions and getting the most efficient lift-off from each step.
- They develop better pace judgment, teaching you not to start races (and speed play) too fast.
- They help the internal systems (muscles, pacing, intuitive connections, and instinctive efficiency adjustments) to work together and become more efficient.
- They fine-tune the components of performance, such as energy sources to the muscle, waste removal, hidden resources to keep going, and so on.
- They develop the mental strength that enables runners to continue running at a good pace even after fatigue sets in.
- They teach you when to keep going and when to avoid damage by stopping.

Pacing in your speed work

Each mile should be run about 30 seconds faster than you want to run in the race itself and should be followed by a walk of about 5 minutes.

DO NOT:

- Run the first 2 to 3 mile repeats too fast
- Go too fast during the first 400 to 800 meters of each mile repeat
- Try to keep up with someone who is faster than you (or who is showing off)
- Over-stride, especially when you start to get tired

Between the mile repeats, walk more than you think you need. This helps your group to stay together and will speed your recovery.

You don't gain anything from running faster than your assigned pace. In fact, you actually hurt your chances of achieving your goal. Even 15 to 20 seconds per mile too fast on the track can lead to extra tiredness and slow recovery. Such fatigue is cumulative and is often carried into the marathon itself. When you reach the last 4 to 6 miles of the marathon, this tiredness will come back to haunt you. Your legs will lack the rebound to maintain or increase speed to the finish.

Also, your pace clock is messed up when you run too fast on the mile repeats. Running 30 seconds faster than your goal pace prepares you to run at that pace in the marathon between the walk breaks. Your muscles and cardiovascular performance system are gearing up to do exactly what they need to do in the actual marathon. By going faster than this, you train yourself to go too fast in the marathon itself; your pace in the early stages tires you quickly and you slow down at the end.

Beware of overexuberance

Start the session, and each mile, slowly. It's always better to go out a little *slower* than you expect to average in the session. This helps the muscles gradually adjust to marathon pace, instead of sending shocks to the system. You're also teaching the energy system to be as efficient as possible.

Adjust for heat and humidity

Even during the extreme heat of summer, you can continue doing speed sessions, but be careful. If you notice yourself or anyone in your group having symptoms of heat disease *(see p. 173)*, stop the session and get medical attention immediately.

On warm days, the best time of the day to do speed sessions is very early in the morning, before the sun rises. When the temperature is above 65 degrees, cut the distance of the reps to 800 meters and run twice as many.

Walk between each mile repeat

It is better to walk between the repetitions to minimize fatigue and recovery. Most runners should walk 5 minutes between each mile repeat and 3 minutes between the 800-meter repeats. Walk more if you feel the need. The extra walking will not reduce the training effect of the speed session. If you have a heart rate monitor, keep walking until the heart rate goes below 70 percent of your maximum heart rate.

Fartlek

Literally, *fartlek* means speed play. It is a free-form method of speed development that can accomplish all of the objectives of interval training and add a mental strengthening component to your training. Used as a substitute for interval training or other speed play, *fartlek* is usually performed on those weekends when you are not making a long run and instead of mile repeats.

Fartleking has several attributes:

- By shifting the use of muscle groups back and forth, you'll develop greater performance capacity. For example, instead of running at the same pace throughout a *fartlek* session, you can use pace running, acceleration, gliding, and speed effort.

- The speed part of *fartlek* should equal the total distance of the number of mile repeats that you would have done on the track, according to the time goal schedule you are following. The speed segments should be at least ¾ mile long but they will give better marathon conditioning if they are 1 mile or longer (1,600 to 3,000 meters).

- As with mile repeats, make sure that you're resting the legs by walking between the speed segments.

To describe a *fartlek*, let's choose a segment that is 1.2 miles long (about 2,000 meters).

1. Start the segment at marathon pace.
2. Several times during the first .6 mile (1,000 meters), put in some acceleration gliders that vary between 100 and 200 meters, each time going back to marathon pace afterward. In other words, start at marathon pace, accelerate for 50 meters, and glide for 50 to 100 meters

before returning to marathon pace. Repeat this sequence two or three times.

3. From about .8 mile to 1.1 mile, shift into speed effort and pick up the pace to about 25 to 30 seconds per mile faster than your marathon goal pace.
4. Glide during the last tenth of a mile.
5. Walk for between 3 and 5 minutes between each *fartlek* segment.
6. Insert walk breaks during each speed segment, as you plan to do during the race.
7. Four of these *fartlek* segments may be done in place of six mile repeats.
8. The three other segments may vary between 1.3 and 1.8 miles (2,200 and 3,000 meters).

Fartlek uses several running modes.

- **Marathon pace** *(see p. 97)*—running smoothly and naturally so that you feel comfortable

- **Accelerations** *(see p. 129)*—picking up the turnover for a short distance, but not expending much effort

- **Gliders** *(see pp. 115–116)*—relaxed and quick turnover motion that follows an acceleration; with practically no effort expended. You're coasting on momentum.

- **Speed effort**—picking up the turnover for a longer distance and running faster than your goal pace; you'll expend some effort doing this, but try to stay smooth and comfortable for the duration of the pick-up.

Mental strength

The mental tenacity you receive from *fartlek* training is enhanced because you are not setting specific limits on where you'll end each segment, each acceleration, each glider. By going beyond artificial barriers, you'll learn to coordinate intuitively the performance demands of the running body with available resources. *Fartlek* desensitizes you to the discomfort and uncertainty of pushing, gliding, and pacing beyond your current limits. Like other training components, *fartlek* must be done regularly to force the systems to work together, to coax out adaptations from the exercising muscle cells, and to develop the intuitive capacity to become more efficient in every way. By pushing through mental and physical barriers at the same time, you'll find yourself continuing to run when you are tired or unmotivated. *Fartlek* develops a sense of focus and resource coordination not found in other forms of training. *(For more on* fartlek, *see Galloway's Book on Running.)*

Marathon rehearsal

During the week, time-goal marathoners can run parts of the shorter runs at marathon pace. As long as the legs, feet, and cardiovascular system have all recovered from the weekend's long run or speed sessions, this race-pace running gives you a chance to lock into the exact cadence clock you need for your goal. After a warm-up, which includes a few acceleration gliders, ease into running 1 to 3 miles at marathon pace. As you get up to speed, you want to feel smooth and efficient. Your goal is to make marathon pace seem normal. Do the walk breaks as planned in your marathon. If the pace and effort levels of hill training and speed sessions are adjusted to your current ability, you should feel at home with marathon pace after a few repetitions. Even one or two of these marathon-goal miles run every other day can help further your pace education.

A walk of between 400 and 800 meters between those paced miles (or a slow jog of 800 meters or more) should leave you completely recovered. It's important to remember that this is not supposed to be a stressful speed session: No significant effort should be required to do each mile and no significant fatigue felt afterward. If it is taking hard work to maintain your marathon pace in these sessions, jog for the rest of the session. Such difficulties mean either that you're just not ready for the chosen pace or that you haven't recovered from the runs of the previous week.

Marathon race form

Using your running muscles continuously in the same way will tire them quickly. If you regularly change your running form modes, even during a mile repeat, you'll allow the calves and hamstrings to relax. Even a slight relaxation, when done regularly, is often enough to infuse a little resilience into the legs. By the end of the speed session, you'll still feel strong, even if you're getting tired, and you'll experience a faster recovery between this exercise session and the next long run or race. This process teaches marathon muscles to automatically shift usage during the 26-mile journey itself.

It's crucial to shift early and shift often. You don't have to go more than 50 to 100 meters when gliding and so on, but you must start early and do it regularly on each mile repeat to get the benefits.

Form modes

• **Race form** About 90 percent of your running in the speed sessions and the marathon will be done using race form. This is a very efficient running motion at a pace that is 30 seconds per mile faster than your marathon goal pace. If you're actually in condition to run the pace you are predicting, little effort is required when running in this mode.

- **Gliding** Every 300 to 600 meters of running at race form, let your feet shift lower to the ground and glide for 30 to 60 meters. When gliding correctly, you'll lose only 1 to 2 meters every 100 meters and you'll find that it takes very little effort, as you use mostly momentum and mechanical efficiency to move. Practice gliding on all of your runs to develop the most efficient motion, using the least effort while moving at the best speed.

- **Efficient rhythm accelerations** ERAs are very short (10- to 20-meter) leg turnovers. While maintaining race form, pick up the rhythm or cadence of your feet and legs. This will gain back the 2 to 3 meters you lost when gliding. Don't lift your knees, don't extend your lower leg out in front of you, and never sprint (that is, run all out). This technique is meant to provide a very short pick-up that shouldn't cause you to huff and puff. The only change to your running form will be an increase in the rhythm of your legs.

- **Shuffling** With your feet low to the ground, maintain a race cadence with very little effort. This comes in handy at water stops, helping you to drink the water instead of drenching your clothes. Shuffling is an alternative to walk breaks at the end of any long run when legs start to cramp.

- **You are the captain** of your running ship and may choose whatever sequence of running modes you like. Here's a suggestion of how to arrange the modes during a mile repeat: Start with race form for 300 to 600 meters, then glide for 50 to 100 meters, return to race form for 200 to 300 meters, put in an ERA for 10 to 20 meters, then glide and ERA, shift back to race form, and glide in.

AFRICANS DO IT

Elite African runners and other world-class runners seldom run more than 200 yards using the same form mode. They're constantly alternating between race form, gliding, shuffling, and ERAs, as they race through the course.

Fun innovations

The greatest benefit of shifting modes is the opportunity to transform what used to be a workout into a playout. Find at least a few ways to divert yourself and/or the members of your speed group and the session becomes an event to look forward to. You're taking an experience that's challenging and rewarding and combining it with incidents of fun generated by the chemistry of individuals. Here are a few suggestions of how various groups have helped speed become playful.

Diversions Brief, improvised skits in which somebody will do something to entertain the others. In planning these, the members of the speed group stay in touch during the week and build a sense of community.

Controversy It takes only two individuals in a group to have different viewpoints on an issue for the whole group to have some fun with it.

Games Even silly children's games such as tag can lighten up the end of a difficult session. Avoid the temptation to overextend your stride length though.

QUESTIONS

"I can't finish a speed session. My legs just can't keep going at the pace needed. What's wrong?"

If you're having trouble maintaining pace on the mile repeats, there are several possibilities:

- Your goal is too ambitious for your current fitness level—adjust to slower repetitions.
- You went out too fast in the first part of the speed session—slow down in the beginning.
- You are still fatigued from other sessions—you need more rest days or easier rest days.
- You need more rest between mile repeats—double the walking between each mile.

"I feel great on the repeat mile sessions and have no trouble running them 40 seconds per mile faster than my goal pace, but my legs don't 'have it' in the marathon itself. Won't running the mile repeats faster help me run faster in the marathon?"

No! You're actually hurting yourself by running the mile repeats faster than your assigned time (30 seconds faster than your goal pace). That pace increase will develop the performance capacity and the pace judgment that are necessary in the marathon. The effort required to go faster than this can keep you tired for many days and compromise the other aspects of your program. Stick with the schedule for your best chance of success.

"Between the mile repeats, I've been jogging instead of walking because I've heard that I'll get in better shape. Is this true?"

No. By walking rather than jogging between the hard repetitions, you won't lose any of the conditioning of that speed session. The extra rest that walking provides will help the legs start recovering from a speed session while you're still doing it. Walking between mile repeats performs the same function as walk breaks during the long run, keeping the running muscles from getting overextended. If you've been running at the assigned pace on the mile repeats, liberal walk breaks between the repeat sessions will allow you to recover within a day or two in most cases.

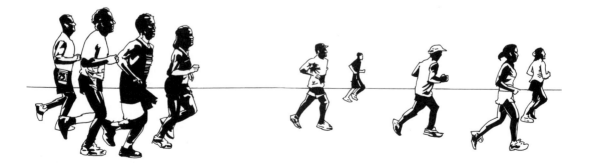

VI FOOD AND FAT BURNING

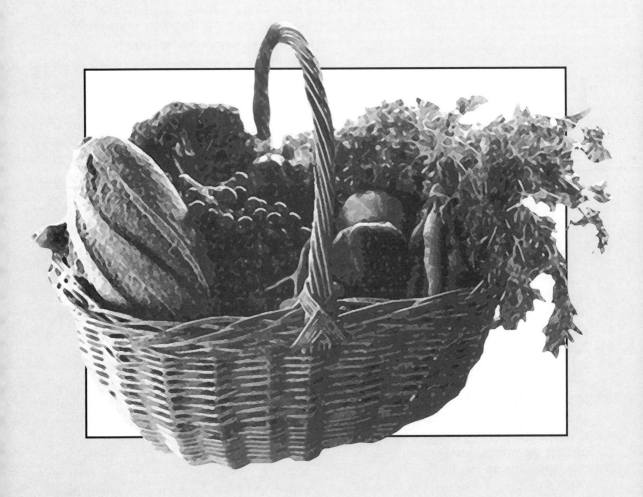

20

FAT BURNING AS A WAY OF LIFE

"After seven marathons in five years, I've lost 35 pounds and kept it off. I must say, however, that I was disappointed that I didn't lose a single pound while training for my first one."

If running is one of the very best ways to burn fat, why then do so few marathoners lose weight—at least in their first campaign? Among the many good answers to this question is that a novice marathoner should plan to arrive at the starting line and then get to the finish line injury-free. The low mileage associated with the training program for this insurance policy will not burn much fat off the body.

Marked dietary changes usually disrupt your metabolism, cause an inconsistent mental focus, and lead to energy surges and withdrawals. Other problems encountered by those who change their diet and train for a marathon at the same time may include stress fractures, nutritional deficiencies, and reductions in blood sugar levels. All can leave you unmotivated to exercise. It's no wonder that we see a lot of dropouts among those who radically change their diets. After crossing that marathon finish line for the first time, you're free to set up a five-year plan for making nutritional changes. *(See p. 40 for a program for fat burning with an expanded schedule of exercise and cross training.)*

In the meantime, let's look into the (unfortunately) expanding world of fat. To better understand how to take it off, we'll look first at how it goes on and the powerful biological instincts that try to keep it in storage. Then we'll focus on the long-term ways of burning it off as a lifestyle. Once you transform yourself into a fat-burning organism, you'll feel better all day long as you burn more fat.

FAT AS FUEL

Our "set point" determines how much fat we store

Humans are lazy. With a primary mission of survival, we are programmed to build up extra fat storage as an insurance policy. For millions of years, this propensity has allowed our ancestors to survive through periods of starvation and sickness. The mechanisms of fat storage, described below, support a well-established principle called "set point," which determines how much we store. *This powerful regulatory mechanism increases your appetite for weeks or months after periods of reduced calorie intake, illness, and even psychological deprivation, all of which deplete fat.* Unfortunately, it does its job too well, leaving you fatter than you were before. Understanding how the set point works as your hedge against starvation is the most important step in learning how to adjust it downward, or at least manage it, for the rest of your life.

What is fat?

When you eat a pat of butter, you might as well inject it onto your thigh or stomach: Dietary fat is deposited directly. Protein and carbohydrates (even sugar) will be converted into fat only when you've consumed too many calories from those sources throughout the day. If you're trying to reduce the fat blanket, it helps to eat complex carbohydrates (baked potatoes, rice, whole grains, and vegetables) and lean sources of protein (legumes, turkey breast, nonfat dairy products, etc.).

Only body fat is used as fuel, not the fat in your diet. It is an excellent energy source, leaving a small amount of waste product, which is easily removed through the increased blood flow of exercise. While stored sugar is limited, you can't run far enough to use up your fat storage. Even a 140-pound person with the unusually low level of 2 percent body fat has hundreds of miles of fuel on board and it is the best fuel for running.

Fat storage differs for men and women

Men tend to store fat on the surface of the body, often on the outside of the stomach area. Most women store fat internally at first. Thousands of pockets between muscle cells are filled up invisibly. Many young women feel that some dramatic change has occurred around the age of 30 when they suddenly start showing accumulations of fat on the outside of their bodies while maintaining the same diet and level of exercise. They've actually been storing fat inside for many years. Once the inner areas are filled, women notice a dramatic change on the outside of their thighs or stomachs, often in less than a year.

How fat accumulates as you get older

By the time humans enter their mid-20s, most have settled into an accustomed level of calorie burning and calorie consumption. Your set point is adjusted for the amount of fat you've accumulated to that point. The set point is programmed to increase your fat accumulation slightly each year. Very slowly, your basal metabolism rate (the calories that are burned each day to keep you alive and doing routine activities) is reduced. But your appetite doesn't decrease very quickly, so most humans consume a few more calories than they need, each week, producing a slow increase in fat accumulation. The internal set point quickly adjusts itself to the higher level of fat and becomes the new set point. Because fat helps one survive a prolonged illness or other major interruption of good health or food intake, increased fat levels are biologically reinforced with each additional year of age.

Diets don't work!

By depriving yourself of food, you can reduce your body fat temporarily as you reduce your metabolism rate and your motivation to exercise. But, as soon as the diet is over, your set-point mechanism unleashes a starvation reflex that keeps you eating until the fat levels are slightly higher than they were before the diet. At the same time, your metabolism rate stays low to help you store fat more quickly. No matter how mentally focused you are, you'll find yourself with more fat on your frame when you mess with that very powerful survival mechanism.

The starvation reflex

Over millions of years, our ancestors withstood regular famines, establishing complex and quick reactions to prepare themselves for even the possibility of food reduction. If you're getting enough food —often enough—your system doesn't feel the need to store fat. But the reflex starts into action when you've waited too long between snacks or meals on any day. The longer you wait to eat, the more you stimulate the fat-depositing enzymes. When you next eat, more of that food will be processed into fat. But that's not all of the bad news. A longer wait between meals increases your appetite, which leads to overeating—during the next meal or over the next few hours. Even if you've eaten three to five times a day but have eaten too few calories for that day's activities, you'll experience an increased appetite during the next 12 to 36 hours.

Psychological starvation

Depriving yourself of food that you dearly love will start a psychological time bomb. You can tell yourself that you'll never eat another doughnut, hamburger, french fry, and so on. You may even be able to abstain for an extended period of time. But at some point in the future, when the food is around and no one else is, your starvation

reflex will gain the upper hand and you'll binge. Over time, the binges will lead you to consume more of that fatty food than you had deprived yourself of during the period of prohibition, and you'll experience a net gain. Moderation is the key.

Burning it off: Regular exercise improves disease resistance

One of the very best and proven ways of readjusting the set point that regulates your appetite to maintain fat accumulation at a certain level is by doing regular endurance exercise. We're not just talking about increased fat burning during exercise. The increased health benefits of regular exercise (enhanced resistance to disease, stronger heart, more efficient cardiovascular system, etc.) give intuitive signals to the body that the risk of long-term health problems has been lowered and there is less need for increased fat levels. A fit 70-year-old, for example, can often fight off disease better and quicker than can an average, not very fit, 30-year-old. Your set-point mechanism seems to have a sensor that intuitively monitors long-term trends in your body. In most cases, the set point is adjusted higher in those in poor health.

Regular running and walking keeps fat off the body, burning off excess calories. Most beginning runners experience some fat burn off, even when their weight stays the same, particularly when their diet is not dramatically increased. If you've consumed more calories than you've burned during a given day, you can literally burn them off with an after-dinner walk or jog. This is particularly helpful if the excess calories on a given day have come from carbohydrates.

Burning fat while you sleep!

Running regularly for more than 45 minutes at a time (even with walk breaks) trains our exercising muscle cells to be fat burners at all times of the night and day. After months of regular distance running, you will have transformed a vast number of running muscle cells into fat burners that prefer fat as a fuel, even when you are sitting around all day or asleep at night. Long runs that exceed 90 minutes, when done every two to three weeks, speed up the transformation of the muscle cells from sugar burners to fat burners.

Sugar-burning produces waste buildup—so slow down!

Fat is the main fuel, but the body also uses another type. Glycogen is the form of sugar that is stored in the muscles for quick energy. Not only is this the fuel that gets us started, but also it sustains us for the first half hour of exercise. Unfortunately, when this form of sugar is used for exercise, it leaves behind a lot of waste product, lactic acid, which causes discomfort. Running even a little too fast at the beginning depletes valuable glycogen quicker as it fills up the muscles and slows them down. This is why many runners don't feel great during the first few miles of a run. The faster the starting pace, the more uncomfortable we feel. Most of this discomfort can be eliminated with a slow start and more frequent or longer early walk breaks—in short, a better warm-up. But more waste is still produced from using up glycogen than is produced when we are burning fat.

The supply of glycogen is very limited, and it is necessary for brain function. A small amount of this fuel is burned every mile, even after you've shifted primarily into fat burning. So it's important on long runs to conserve this resource by keeping the pace slow from the beginning. When supplies run low, your body will hold back enough to keep the brain, your most crucial organ, functioning and, for the rest of your energy needs, force a breakdown of fat and protein—a very uncomfortable process. You can avoid this by gradually increasing your distance, by putting in more walk breaks from the beginning, and by running at least three days a week; being regular is important.

After running 45 minutes, you'll be burning mostly fat

By starting at a slow pace and taking walk breaks as needed, you can lower your exertion level enough to stay in the fat-burning zone for an extended time. This conserves glycogen for later use as you burn off the extra blanket around your stomach or thighs. From 15–45 minutes, your muscles gradually shift into fat-burning

Your body does not believe that you're really going out on a distance run until you keep moving forward for more than a quarter hour. At this point, you begin to break down body fat for fuel (dietary fat is converted directly into body fat and is not burned for energy). It takes some work to break down the "excess baggage" on your body into free fatty acids and triglycerides that can keep you running mile after mile. If you continue exercising longer than about 15 minutes at a pace that is within your capacity, you start shifting into fat-burning. As your exercise continues past the quarter-hour mark, you start a transition into fat-burning as long as you continue to exercise at a level of exertion that is within your capacity.

HOT TIP FOR BURNING FAT

Increase the length of all your runs to more than 45 minutes.

Training your muscles to burn fat

Those who are not in shape for endurance activity must train their muscles to burn fat. Beginning exercisers may have to limit their exercise to walking until they can work up to an hour or more of continuous activity. Instead of walk breaks, some completely out-of-shape beginners may need to take 1- to 2-minute "sit down" breaks every 5 to 8 minutes to stay in the fat-burning zone. After a few weeks, however, most of those novices can accomplish continuous 45- to 60-minute walks at a steady pace. At that point, they may increase the walking distance or hold the distance steady and add jogging breaks *(see box on p. 138)*. Some people take longer to progress. Be patient.

The adaptation to fat burning is more difficult for those who've done little or no exercise before. If you're in this category, do more walking and stick with it. The fat-burning process works for you the same as it does for world-class athletes. You may not notice it for a while because the changes are going on inside the muscle cells. Keep telling yourself "I'm becoming a fat-burning furnace" because you are!

Aerobic exercise

Fast anaerobic exercise burns sugar; slow aerobic exercise burns fat Fat in the muscle cells can be burned only when there's an adequate supply of oxygen. This is aerobic exercise: exertion that is done at an easy enough pace so that the blood can provide all of the oxygen needed by the muscles. As soon as you increase the pace beyond your current capacity or go farther than your muscles are trained to go, the muscles can't get enough oxygen to burn fat and so they shift back to the readily available but inefficient energy source, glycogen. Your exercise is now anaerobic, meaning that the muscles aren't getting enough oxygen. The longer and faster you run anaerobically, the worse you'll feel and the sooner you'll quit because of the accumulation of lactic acid. (For a more detailed explanation of this process, see *Galloway's Book on Running*.)

Walk breaks and a slow pace at the start keep you in the fat-burning zone longer. If you're used to running for 5 miles (at 12 minutes per mile) with no walk breaks, try slowing down to run at between 14 and 16 minutes per mile. This will reduce your level of exertion so that you can run for 6 to 8 miles while feeling the same way you felt after 5 miles. When you add a 1-minute walk break every 1–3 minutes, you can push the wall back to between 7 and 10 miles while feeling as though you covered only about half that distance. It's always better to increase your mileage gradually, so I recommend that you make this type of increase over several runs. The slower running with walk breaks will allow you to extend the distance with little or no risk of injury or over-fatigue. The extra mileage means that you are burning more calories and fat.

The continuous movement of the body during long, slow runs and walks (lasting at least 45 minutes) mobilizes an incredible number of muscle cells in the legs, back, butt, and related areas. By slowly covering several miles, three times a week, this network of muscles specializes in the work that can keep moving the body in the most efficient way. Because fat is the most efficient and abundant fuel, the muscles will adapt to become fat burners if this run is done regularly enough.

Stoking your fat-burning furnace

By slowing down enough to break the 45-minute barrier and exercise for longer periods, you show your body that you're serious about endurance. It responds by converting the formerly sugar-burning cells into fat burners. The minimum necessary is one session longer than 45 minutes per week, but the process is accelerated by exercising for more than 90 minutes once every two weeks. As the long-run distance increases significantly in a marathon (or half-marathon) program, you force more and more cells into the more efficient mode of fat metabolism and keep them there. To maintain the capacity of your expanding fat furnace, you'll need at least two other 30-minute sessions a week. If each of these can be increased to at least 45 minutes, you'll improve the adaptation. As always, it's better to slow down from the beginning of exercise so that you'll feel better, be more motivated to continue, and go further.

Burning fat in the office and while you sleep

Running and walking elevate your core body temperature. Many experts believe that this produces a healthy "fever" that often kills off infections before they cause colds or worse. But the greater your blanket of body fat, the more heat you'll retain, which can lead to excessive fluid loss through sweating. Your body's temperature control mechanism will try to reduce this source of stress if you run regularly. After months of regular long runs, you'll slowly burn off the blanket, reducing your set point, and therefore your body fat, if you're not significantly increasing calorie intake.

As more of the muscle cells adapt to fat metabolism through training, you'll be burning more fat throughout the day. Once they've run enough long runs, regularly, even sedentary office workers will burn fat while sitting in their offices or on the couch at night. Endurance-trained fat-burning cells will choose more fat as their fuel even while you are asleep. Then, in the "battle of the bulge," you'll be able to enlist as your soldiers thousands of cells gobbling fat all day and all night.

The virtue of patience

We Americans often want changes to occur too rapidly. If a little exercise burns x amount of fat, we are tempted to log twice as many miles to double the rate. This doesn't work. By adding too much distance too soon, you'll get tired or injured, and be forced to stop exercising or to cut back dramatically. Even worse is the possibility that you'll get mentally burned out. If you continue to run slowly and increase your total weekly mileage by no more than 10 percent, you'll reduce chances of injury and burn-out to almost nothing.

The biggest mistake runners make is to start a run too hard, too fast. This is so easy to do because it usually doesn't *feel* too hard, but 6 to 10 minutes later you're wishing that you were finished. By forcing yourself to start much more slowly than you want, you'll get a stream of benefits, speed your entry into the fat-burning zone and set yourself up for more enjoyment later.

Walk breaks can help you burn off 10 pounds of fat!

To show you why it's better to go slowly, let's look at the math in the table at right. Continuous running (whether slow or fast) burns about 100 calories per mile. If you're walking normally, you're burning about 50 calories per mile. Even if you're running for 2 minutes and walking for 1 minute, you're closer to the running side of the continuum, burning about 80 calories per mile. Let us suppose, then, that you're running 5 miles on four days a week. If you slowed down and took a 1-minute walk break for every 3 minutes of running, you'd feel about the same, after covering 8 miles, as you would feel if you'd run 5 miles continuously. Here's the math:

8 miles (85 calories per mile = 680 calories per run)

5 miles (100 calories per mile = 500 calories per run)

That's an increase of 180 calories per run.

In one year, your walk breaks will enable you to burn off an extra 10 pounds of fat!

ENERGIZING TIP

Eat before you really get hungry.

BURN CALORIES WHILE WALKING

Calories per mile	Pace
50	Recreational walking
55	4–5 minutes walking; 1 minute jogging
60	3–4 minutes walking; 1 minute jogging
65	2 minutes walking; 1 minute jogging
70	1 minute walking; 1 minute jogging
75	Racewalking
75	2 minutes jogging; 2 minutes walking
80	2 minutes jogging; 1 minute walking
85	3 minutes jogging; 1 minute walking
90	4–5 minutes jogging; 1 minute walking
95	6–7 minutes jogging; 1 minute walking
90	8–9 minutes jogging; 1 minute walking
100	Running continuously

Why didn't I lose weight during my marathon programs?

Don't use the scales as your gauge of fat loss. You've probably lost fat while training, even though your weight stays the same. Although fat is burned during your runs, other physiological changes will increase your body weight in a healthy way, helping you to improve your performance. More water and glycogen are stored in the muscle cells so that you can stay cooler and maintain your levels of energy during exercise. Your blood volume also increases when you do regular endurance running and walking so the exercising muscles are more easily supplied with oxygen and nutrients. All three of these changes increase body weight, but in a good way, preparing you for easier and better running.

Don't diet while training for a marathon

A four- to six-month endurance program produces enough challenges to your life-style without the additional stress of a diet change. To accomplish your goal of run-ning a marathon, you need a steady flow of energy. When you're strenuously training while on a diet, the energy supply is often interrupted, resulting in low motivation and feelings of discouragement during and after runs.

When you are gearing up the body to go 26 miles, I want you to focus on four items:

1. Incorporating regular endurance exer-cise into your lifestyle
2. Building the endurance necessary to go the distance
3. Learning how to enjoy the process so you'll want to do it again
4. Staying injury-free

If you try to change your diet during this mission, you're very likely to suffer from confused priorities. It's so easy to think that you're eating healthier foods while you omit certain nutrients needed for performance. Unfortunately, the loss of these nutritional building blocks isn't noticed until weeks or months later when you're dragging around—unmotivated to exercise.

Unless you had nutritional problems before the program started, stick with the diet that you've been using. Certainly it's okay to divide up your food into more small meals a day and to reduce your fat intake a little, but don't make any radical changes. If you feel that you have some nutritional problems at any time, see a sports nutri-tionist, preferably one who has had success in working with long-distance runners. During a marathon program it's okay to say "I'm starting my diet later"—after the marathon.

21 HOW YOU EAT DETERMINES HOW GOOD YOU FEEL

A successful eating plan is one that has all the essential nutrients, allows you to maintain a good energy level for exercise and for daily activities, and maintain the body fat level with which you feel comfortable. For fat-level management, you must understand the principles of your set point and be honest with yourself. This means balancing what you want to look like with the type of eating plan you're willing to follow, not for a month or so, but as a lifestyle. Most successful dietary changes are small ones that allow you to feel good all day long so you can exercise and burn off the pounds of fat you want to lose.

The primary purpose of this chapter is to help you set up an eating plan that will give you sufficient energy for your daily activities as well as marathon training. Fat burning should be a longer-term activity and integrated into your lifestyle, taking a back seat to the establishment of exercise as the prime mover in your personal wellness program. Exercise burns the fat, is the furnace that keeps it off, and gives you the good attitude and the reason to continue working toward your goal. Just knowing that you're burning it off gives purpose to your dietary changes. But it works both

ways. Your eating plan can give you the energy you need to be motivated to exercise as it delivers the nutrients for muscle exertion and repair. Most runners find that only a few changes in eating frequency and food choices make the difference in keeping off the baggage that they worked so hard to get rid of.

The point of eating is to acquire the essential nutrients with a steady metabolism boost so that you can maintain a motivational level of blood sugar to do all of life's activities. Your energy level is somewhat determined by what you eat and significantly influenced by how much and how often you eat.

Eating all day long

Yes, it's better for fat control and your energy level if you eat every hour and a half. Our digestion system was designed for grazing: Taking in modest amounts of food all day long. Each time we eat, even small amounts, our digestive system gears up to process the nutrients and dispose of the bulk. This means that you're burning calories for an extended period beyond the eating of the snack—in order to digest the food.

GOOD NUTRITION
IN A NUTSHELL

- It's important to reduce dietary fat over time.
- It's best to get your nutrients mostly in food.
- A variety of foods, including fresh fruit and vegetables, will deliver nutrients well.
- It's better to eat seven to nine small meals a day rather than two or three bigger ones.
- Try to make each meal consist mostly of complex carbohydrates balanced with some protein and a little fat.
- Most women and some men tend to have an iron deficiency and should take supplements.
- A quality vitamin supplement can help in preventing certain types of cancer.
- Change your diet over three to five years, five being better than three.

LOSE A LITTLE HERE . . . A LITTLE THERE

Fat loss in a year (lbs.)	Method
Up to 10	Eating the same foods in the same quantity but eating frequently, between eight and ten times a day instead of three or fewer.
5–20	Getting out of your chair at work or off the couch at home several times a day to increase your metabolism
1–3	Doing more of your runs because of a motivational level of blood sugar
1–3	Parking 100 meters further away on each trip to the supermarket
2–5	Going farther on numerous runs because your blood sugar level is higher
2–5	Substituting a baked potato for a large serving of fries once a week
2–5	Walking around the block (sometimes twice) after supper

The starvation reflex kicks into depositing fat when your metabolism slows down. Even if you wait 3 hours to eat, you'll increase the fat-depositing enzymes so that more of the next meal becomes fat. To prevent starvation, you have an intuitive mechanism that conserves resources and adds fat to the body if you're not grazing regularly. The longer you go without food, the more your metabolism will shut down into a fasting or low level of energy. If you're not eating enough food, "metabolism control" will cut your flow of energy so that you don't burn up your reserves. The longer you fast, the more likely you will want to be sedentary and resist moving around. So if you're trying to exercise in the afternoon, 5 hours after your last meal or snack, your metabolism controller will probably be steering you toward the couch instead of the track or trail.

A small to moderate snack will increase your metabolism significantly and can be processed efficiently. A big meal will take a while to process. Your metabolism gears up to process it, but so many resources are needed (especially blood supply) that your body wants to shut down other activities. This is why you feel sleepy and unmotivated about half an hour after a big meal.

> Even an energy bar, eaten, with a glass of water, an hour before exercise will raise your blood sugar to workout motivation levels. It's still better, however, to eat snacks all day long, instead of waiting until you feel extremely hungry.

What you eat makes a difference

A good balance of fresh, complex carbohydrates along with some protein and a little fat will leave you satisfied for an extended period after eating. Too much food, too much sugar and starch, and too much fat in a meal will lead to fat accumulation.

Carbohydrates Carbohydrates give you the energy you need in a form the body can easily use. Complex carbohydrates (such as vegetables, fruits, whole grain products, legumes, etc.) have fiber and various other nutrients neatly packaged with the energy. They keep you satisfied for longer because it takes the body a longer time to process them. Simple carbohydrates (sugar, starch, etc.) are broken down so fast that you can consume a great quantity of calories without feeling satisfied. Excess calories that accumulate during a day are processed into fat if, after several hours, they haven't been needed for energy.

Fat Fat is deposited directly on your body. A little fat in each snack or meal will keep you from being hungry for a longer period. But once the fat content exceeds about 25 percent of the calories, particularly in a meal, you'll be storing significant quantities. Fat slows down digestion, so you'll be more uncomfortable if you want to run too soon after eating. The more fat you eat, the more lethargic you'll feel.

Eating fat after exercise also slows down your restocking of glycogen. A high-carbohydrate meal with 20% of the calories in protein within 30 minutes after a run will help you restock the vital energy supply you need for the first 15 to 30 minutes of exercise. When too much fat is consumed, the glycogen is not replenished and you don't feel very good as you start each successive run.

Sugar and starch Sugar and starch are simple carbohydrates and are processed so quickly that you usually get hungry before you've even had a chance to burn them off. As we tend to follow our hunger pangs, meals overloaded with sugar and starch almost always lead us to consume more calories in a 24-hour period than we are burning off. Excess calories are transformed into body fat. Small quantities of simple carbohydrates are okay —especially if they are in a food that you dearly love. Don't prevent yourself from eating that piece of pizza; just enforce the one-slice rule.

Protein Protein is the building block of our muscles. We need some each day to replace the normal wear and tear of our muscles and other tissue. By eating some protein with each of your snacks, you'll prolong your feeling of satisfaction—extending the time before you feel hungry. You can certainly eat too much protein. If your total consumption of calories during a day is more than you've burned up, the excess will be converted into fat—whether the surplus comes from carbohydrates, protein, fat or all three. Too much protein in the diet can cause other health problems. Most nutritionists I've interviewed have told me that a steady diet in which 30 percent or more consists of protein can lead to kidney damage.

Fiber Fiber will also keep you from getting hungry for a while. Many types of soluble fiber, such as oat bran, coat the lining of the stomach, slowing down the release of sugars into the bloodstream. I've found that energy bars, which have a very effective form of soluble fiber, keep me from getting hungry for about twice as long as do

other energy bars with less fiber. Practically any fiber that is in a food will increase the feeling of satisfaction. A baked potato, for example, leaves me satisfied for about three times as long as an apple does, although each has the same number of calories. The fiber in a baked potato is much more complex than that in apples, and the latter have much more sugar.

Vitamins and minerals A variety of fresh fruits and vegetables together with sources of lean protein will usually give you more nutrients than you need. But as an insurance policy, I recommend a good "one-a-day"-type vitamin. Some good research points to the possibility of cancer reduction if you take vitamin C (500 mg), and vitamins D and E (400 iu) every day. Other research shows that deficiency of the B complex can encourage heart disease through the buildup of plaque. Vitamin C definitely speeds up the healing process. Women who exercise regularly tend to be deficient in iron and sometimes in calcium.

Alcohol Alcohol is a central nervous system depressant, and is almost certain to lower your performance if consumed within about 12 hours of exercise. The more you drink, the longer the depressing effect lasts. Alcohol also dehydrates you. It's not a good idea to drink the night before a long run, fast run, or a race.

Caffeine Caffeine is a central nervous system stimulant that can enhance the performance and enjoyment of exercise. But a few individuals should not take it. Those, for example, who have problems with an irregular heartbeat shouldn't be drinking coffee. If you suspect that you might have problems with caffeine, check with your doctor or a sports nutritionist.

I dearly enjoy my cup of coffee before my run. It not only raises my awareness, concentration and motivation, but also seems to get the right brain working its intuitive magic, cranking out creative thoughts. Caffeine stimulates an early breakdown of your body fat into free fatty acids and triglycerides, substances that can be burned as fuel. There's also good evidence that a cup of coffee about an hour before exercise improves your endurance. But you will lose about half the water in a cup of coffee or in a diet cola. This means that only half of the fluid is available for absorption. A cup of coffee before a race is fine if you're accustomed to doing this before running, but three cups or more are not.

Regulating the appetite

Over the course of a month we tend to eat the number of calories that we burn up, that rate being controlled by our internal set-point mechanism. When the mechanism senses that we're engaging the starvation reflex, it will trigger more hunger and we'll eat more calories than we're burning,

producing a weight gain. By eating small meals every few hours, exercising regularly, eating complex carbohydrates, and so on, we'll tend to stay the same or burn off more calories than we've consumed. This results in fat reduction. Simple sugars and starches just slide through with no discount, producing surplus calories that are converted into body fat. Even if you eat too many calories in carbohydrates and protein, you can still go out for a walk or jog and burn them off—another way to gain control over your weight and fat level.

The best time for reloading after exercise is within 30 minutes of finishing your run. But you can still get reload benefits for the next 2 hours. Be sure to drink water or other fluids (except those containing caffeine or alcohol) during the reloading process. By drinking fluids and eating some high-quality carbohydrate snack (enhanced by adding about 20 percent protein by calorie count), you can maximize glycogen reloading and will feel better and stronger during your next run.

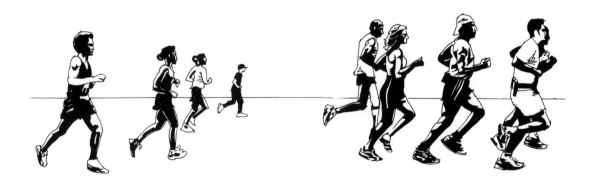

PUTTING IT ALL ON THE TABLE

Here's an exercise that will help you lose up to ten pounds a year without reducing the amount of food you eat or increasing the amount of exercise you take.

1. On a piece of paper, write down all the food you eat in a week. Collect this information by carrying a journal with you and recording everything you eat, day by day. Note the food and the amount (you may need a tiny gram scale). When possible, get the recipe and/or the nutrient breakdown, that is, the number of calories from fat, protein, and carbohydrates. (Libraries and bookstores carry publications of tables giving this sort of information, or use a website such as www.fitday.com.)

2. Once you have your weekly totals, imagine that you're putting all of this food on a table. It may take a big table. You'll probably be surprised at your findings.

3. List each food and the total the number of grams or ounces of it that you have consumed.

4. Now for the fun! Arrange the total into about 60 or 70 small meals so that you've used up everything. Try to combine the foods so that you have some fat (10 to 20 percent of the calories), some protein (10 to 25 percent of the calories), and the rest carbohydrates in each meal. Also, try to have some fiber in each meal. You'll have some larger meals every day and lots of small ones.

5. Once you get accustomed to combining foods, you'll discover the proportions of fat, protein, and fiber that keep you satisfied and the quantities of carbohydrates that give you energy. Don't use someone else's combinations because each of us responds differently to specific foods.

6. For help with your diet, consult a sports nutritionist. Good reference books are *The Sports Nutrition Handbook* by Nancy Clark, MS, RD and *A Woman's Guide to Fatburning* by Jeff and Barbara Galloway.

LOWFAT FOODS THAT INCREASE SATISFACTION

Protein

Nonfat or lowfat chicken breasts (frozen)

Nonfat or lowfat deli turkey

Egg whites

Soy burgers

Some white fish (many fish have a high fat content)

Vegetables

Most cooked vegetables

Salads

Coleslaw with nonfat mayonnaise

Soup—in cans or dry mix in a cup

Filler foods

Baked potatoes

Brown rice (feel satisfied longer)

White rice

Cereals

Grape-Nuts can be added to many snacks to prolong satisfaction

Oatmeal with fruit or in a smoothie

Oat bran can be added to drinks, soup, pancakes, muffins, and bread

Fruits

Smoothies with oat bran

Baked goods

Whole grain or crusty and fibrous bread

Small meals

Oat bran pancakes or waffles with a smoothie topping (bananas, strawberries and orange juice)

Grape-Nuts with a banana, grapes, or sliced apples

Whole grain or oat bran bagel with lowfat or fat-free cream cheese

Baked potato (skin and all), fat-free cream cheese, low or nonfat coleslaw

Turkey breast or ground turkey burgers with vegetable of choice

Chicken breast with rice, vegetables, whole grain breads

Smoothie: combinations of between one and three varieties of any fruit with fruit juice. For example, combine a banana with frozen strawberries, orange juice concentrate, yogurt, and oat bran, if desired.

Energy bars: several different flavors

Remember to drink water with every snack.

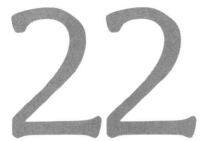

22 BOOSTING BLOOD SUGAR— & MOTIVATION

"Eating during my marathon allowed me to mentally feel great after the marathon and party that evening."

The level of sugar in your blood determines your feeling of well-being. If the blood sugar level (BSL) is in a good, normal range, you can concentrate better, feel more motivated, and there'll be fewer negative messages coming from your left brain. When you let the BSL get too low, you'll get hungry, feel drowsy, lose your focus, and be susceptible to quitting early.

Most folks wake up in the morning with a BSL that is stable, although slightly low. Snacks or meals that include complex carbohydrates, protein, and a little fat will elevate the level slightly and still keep it stable. Foods that are too high in sugar (or other simple carbohydrates) will boost the sugar level too high, too quickly.

MAINTAINING BSL

- Snack every 2 hours.
- Each snack should have complex carbohydrates, protein (15–25% of the calories) and fat (10–20% of the calories).
- Drink 6–8 oz. of water with each snack.

During my first 70 or so marathons, I didn't eat anything. After each of them, my blood sugar level was so low that I hardly enjoyed the exhilaration of even the better ones. I thought that low blood sugar was a given, that the level would crash regardless of what I did on all runs longer than 20 miles. Even on my best marathons, I finished feeling exhausted, unmotivated, unable to concentrate very well, and very hungry but often nauseous. A good nap usually turned into a long evening's hibernation. The vitality wasn't in my legs or spirit the next morning—even after some 12 hours of sleep. Then I learned that you can not only feel good during the latter stages of a marathon but also have a good attitude all evening if you make sure that your blood sugar level doesn't get too low.

The blood sugar challenge

When you run farther than about 12 miles, your blood sugar is going to diminish. If you do nothing about it, you may feel depressed at the end of the marathon. Yet, it takes only a small amount of carbohydrates to maintain a stable level of blood sugar.

147

When the BSL gets too high, your monitoring system automatically secretes insulin, which counteracts the rise and reduces the level to a point that is lower than it was before you ate the snack. In addition, insulin processes the extra sugar into body fat.

A low BSL puts a major stress on your system and activates a stream of negative messages from the left side of your brain. "Why am I doing this?" "Slow down and I'll feel better," "If I just stop, I'll feel great." You can often stop these messages completely within half an hour or less. Just eat an energy bar or another energy-boosting snack, choosing foods that will regulate the rise of the BSL and keep it in bounds.

- Choose complex carbohydrates—baked potatoes, rice (especially brown rice), lowfat whole grain breads, or whole grain pasta with lowfat sauces—rather than sugar foods.

- Combine complex carbohydrates with a modest amount of protein. For example, eat a sandwich made of two thick pieces of whole grain bread or a bagel spread with mustard or nonfat cream cheese and filled with a slice or two of lowfat turkey breast.

- The soluble fiber in snacks such as energy bars will coat the lining of the stomach and keep the BSL from rising to the level that will trigger an insulin release. It will also slow down the release of sugars in the food over an extended period of time.

A sign of middle age

Some people, after the age of 35, when they experience hypoglycemia or symptoms of low blood sugar for the first time in their lives, look on it as another betrayal of the body. Relax, this is a common occurrence. More reassuring is the realization that you can do something about it: *Just eat often enough.* You may not, for instance, feel like exercising in the afternoon because it's been too long since you've had a snack. As the time increases between significant snacks of food, your BSL drops and so does your motivation, concentration, and attitude.

The importance of breakfast

Your BSL is best maintained by eating a modest breakfast and then a series of small snacks all day long. By eating a small or modest amount before you get hungry, you'll avoid the starvation reflex, which leads to overeating.

Breakfast should give you a sustained feeling of well-being throughout the morning and reduces the chance of a significant drop in BSL. By eating lowfat snacks (such as pretzels, bagels, energy bars) at the first sign of a slight hunger or BSL drop, you'll maintain your energy, mental concentration, and attitude. Without some breakfast, you'll probably get behind in the blood sugar race, staying hungry all day and overeating at some point. But, you don't have to eat a big breakfast. Any of the following will work.

Sample breakfasts

- One or two bagels, fat-free cream cheese, and fruit

- One or two bowls of whole-grain cereal (like Grape-Nuts), with skim milk, and two pieces of toast with light jam

- One bowl of oatmeal, oat bran, or other hot cereal, two pieces of toast, juice

- Two egg-substitute eggs (or four egg whites), toast or bagel, juice

- Four to eight ounces of fat-free yogurt, oat bran, Grape-Nuts, and fruit cocktail or juice

Increasing the long run and managing your BSL

By gradually increasing the length of your long run (with walk breaks), you'll push back the threshold of a blood sugar crash. As the muscles become better fat burners, they make many adaptations that increase the efficiency of each use of glycogen. This reduces the quantity of glycogen needed for any use—long run, daily activity, and so on—so that there is more glycogen available to you later to maintain your BSL at a higher level for a greater time and distance. As you extend your endurance barriers, you'll go further before experiencing the discomfort of low blood sugar. Your energy system uses glycogen more efficiently and delivers a better quality of fuel at the same time.

Long runs also stimulate the exercising muscles to store more glycogen. By the time you've increased your long run to 20 miles and more, you're not only using less glycogen per mile, but you also have a greater deposit in your bank. The significant improvement in the storage, shifting of supplies, and consumption of glycogen is a prime example of how the human organism is designed to improve when faced with a series of challenges.

Blood sugar boosters

Even if your BSL is ideal at the beginning of a run, it is certain to be dramatically reduced as you push your limits beyond 15 miles (and many runners experience the "crash" before this). Almost everyone will suffer low blood sugar at the end of long runs if he or she does not eat quality carbohydrate snacks before the start and during the second half.

To boost blood sugar levels most runners need to consume between 30 and 40 calories every 1–2 miles during a long run (when they are running more than 15 miles) to keep their BSL sustained.

- Sugar foods are best—gels, hard candy, Gummi Bears, etc.
- If the food is a solid, an energy bar for instance, be sure to drink at least two ounces of water for every 40 calories you are consuming,
- Cut solid foods up into small pieces so that they are easier to consume during the long run and drink some water with each piece
- Test your eating routine during long runs to find the right time sequence, quantity, etc. for you.

Energy foods

Many foods are advertised as sports energizers. Some of the claims are inflated. First, determine what you need from the snack. Next, with the help of knowledgeable running friends, sports nutritionists, or trustworthy running store staff, evaluate the possible products. Then, try several types on long and short runs and choose one or two to consider for the marathon itself. Use your chosen foods on as many runs as possible before the marathon.

You and your digestive tract can learn to like just about anything. Don't give up on a food because it doesn't taste good at first or doesn't seem to work for you the first time. Take small amounts of the food with water at first. Over time, you can increase the amount of the food as your systems learn to digest and use it.

Energy bars

These are high-carbohydrate foods with soluble fiber (energy bars and related products). Supplying a moderate boost of energy, these products usually deliver a good BSL for an extended period. Be sure to check the label of the product you choose to ensure that it is low in fat. (Fat calories should comprise less than 10 percent of the total calories. Fat takes longer to be digested and it is more likely that it will make you lethargic instead of energetic.)

Eat a portion about 1 hour before the run and pieces of the product throughout the second half of the run—always with water.

Energy gels

These are the little soft packets of thick, sweet high-carbohydrate, paste-like products. They usually deliver a stronger BSL boost at first, which wears off after several minutes. Read and follow the directions on the package, and try them out extensively in training runs. Because they are somewhat liquid, they get into the blood stream quicker than bar products do, but you should drink water with each packet, if available. Once you start taking these, you must continue consuming them until the end of the run to avoid a sudden drop in your BSL. *Note:* Nausea may occur when taking the whole packet. I suggest a third to a quarter every 1–2 miles.

Sports drinks

These are beverages with sugar and electrolytes and, while they can be an excellent fluid replacement before and after training runs, the electrolyte beverages tend to send the BSL into a rollercoaster ride when taken in the marathon itself. Without a substance such as soluble fiber to slow down the absorption of the sugar and maintain the level, you can easily encourage an insulin reaction by drinking them regularly. If you are desperate and feel the need to drink some of these products, dilute them with water.

I have been impressed with the research behind Accelerade, an Endurox product, which contains 20% of its calories in protein. As with other foods, if you plan to use them in the marathon, practice taking them on long runs. *Note:* Because many runners are nauseous when taking sports drinks, I suggest using water with a blood sugar booster during long runs.

Concentrated carbohydrate fluids

There are several fluids on the market that offer large quantities of carbohydrates in a small bottle. Similar to syrup, these fluids take a while to digest and require fluid from your body to do so. As they tend to dehydrate you, they are not recommended for drinking either the day before, the morning before, or during the marathon itself (or during comparable times in training runs). Their concentration will often cause fat accumulation because the fluid goes through your digestive system so quickly that you're hungry again before you've had a chance to burn off the significant number of calories they supply.

Hard candies and Gummi Bears

Among the most reliable boosters are Gummi Bears and small, inexpensive hard candies. Each supplies so few total calories that an insulin response is unlikely. If you start eating one or two about every mile after about 4–6 miles, you will gain some BSL boost. It's always better to drink water at every stop when taking these candies. As they have no soluble fiber, keep taking them. Unlike the bar products, sugar candies don't provide a long-lasting boost.

23 THE MARATHON DIET

"At first I had stomach trouble on most of my runs. Then I wrote down what I ate the day before and eliminated the problems. I almost never have stomach problems now."

Food for energy and muscle

If you want to know which pill or snack you can eat to send you zooming to top performance, then get another book. I believe that the most important elements for a successful marathon are steady training with adequate rest. Food will give you energy to train and the raw material to rebuild muscle. North Americans tend to eat a lot of junk food, but they generally get enough nutrients during a six-month period to train for and complete a marathon without incident. If your diet is deficient when you walk to the starting line, it's too late to do anything about it.

Train your stomach for the marathon

Just as you must train your legs to go the distance, you must fine-tune your digestive system to deliver the nutrients under the stress of long runs. In training, you'll steadily eliminate (or adjust the intake of) foods that cause problems. You want to get into a routine, knowing exactly what to eat, when to eat it, how much to drink with it, etc. If you refine this routine during your series of long runs, you'll reduce the chance of problems in the marathon to almost nothing.

Eliminate problem foods

A variety of foods is great for overall nutrition, but your diet immediately before a marathon will be limited. Analyze your eating the day before and the morning of long runs. Over the months, eliminate foods that cause problems. Realize that it may have been the quantity. It's better to eat too little than to eat too much. But don't starve yourself. Continue to eat small meals or snacks (which you know will be digested quickly) all day long and into the evening.

To establish a useful pattern, start by making notes of your diet, using a notebook that you can review before your next long run. Note what you ate, how much, and at what time, and also note what fluids, if any, you consumed with it. As you determine the right quantities and timetable, you'll gain control over how you feel the day before and the morning of the long run or marathon.

Everyone should practice "eating on the run." During their mile repeat sessions, time-goal runners will also benefit from eating the booster snack they plan to use in the marathon. This not only prepares the stomach for the marathon, but also the boost will help you get through the speed session and recover faster.

Fluids

Drink non-dehydrating fluids regularly, choosing water, orange juice, or a sports drink. But don't overdo it. When I hear sloshing in my stomach or feel that my stomach is loaded with water, I don't drink for a while. When the sloshing sound goes away, I resume drinking.

If your sodium levels are low and you continue to drink beyond the point of being well hydrated, you may suffer a potentially serious health problem called hyponatremia, or water intoxication. This condition is a life-threatening disruption of the necessary flow of fluids during exercise. It happens rarely, but can be aggravated if you are on a restricted diet, are sick, or taking medications. Experts recommend no more that 20 oz. of fluid per hour.

Sports drinks and the days before and after

Sports drinks are electrolyte beverages that may be used to top off your fluid levels and, to some extent, your glycogen levels. I recommend a maximum of one quart of your favorite sports drink, consumed in increments over the course of the day before and the day after a long run.

Electrolyte beverages (sports drinks) can cause problems on long runs and marathons. The sugar in the drinks overloads the digestive system and slows down the absorption of water, which the body needs greatly. Many runners who use sports drinks in marathons suffer from nausea during the second half—caused by the residue of sports drink fluid which stays in the stomach.

Much of the research on sports drinks was done on cyclists and doesn't apply to runners. In running, the digestive system slows down dramatically and can shut down completely. Because cycling is not stressful enough to shut down digestion, sports drinks can be absorbed. The most impressive research I've seen from sports drinks has been shown by Accelerade.

Caffeine

If you are used to drinking coffee before running, there's no reason not to have one cup before a long run or marathon. Caffeine is a central nervous system stimulant that helps to get your mind and body up to speed from the beginning of a run. It promotes an early breakdown of body fat and has been shown to increase endurance capacity. And, yes, it can get one important personal detail taken care of early so that you don't have to spend time in the portajohn before the race (or wish you could).

Follow the diet that got you here

You may be tempted, after walking through a pre-race expo, to try one of the "miracle foods" that you hear about there. Don't do it! Even if a food is the best in its category, it may cause some significant problems if you haven't used it before. You're going to feel somewhat nervous and stressed and it doesn't take much of a nutritional change to produce intestinal misery.

JEFF GALLOWAY'S EATING COUNTDOWN

The following is the most I would ever eat before a marathon. Usually, I leave out some of the items. This is not meant to be a suggestion for what you should eat—set the schedule that works best for you. When you drink, remember to adhere to the sloshing rule.

The day before a long run or the marathon:

9:00 a.m.	Cereal or bagel with lowfat cream cheese, coffee or tea Drink 8 ounces of water or orange juice or a sports drink
10:30 a.m.	An energy bar or whole grain bagel or baked potato with nonfat coleslaw Drink 8 ounces of water or sports drink
12:00 noon	A grilled chicken sandwich or sliced turkey breast on whole grain bread, steamed broccoli or spinach salad Drink 8 ounces of water or sports drink
1:30–2:00 p.m.	An energy bar or cereal or a baked potato with nonfat sour cream Drink 8 ounces of water or sports drink
3:30–4:00 p.m.	A grilled chicken sandwich or turkey breast burrito with pinto beans and sliced tomatoes; an energy bar Drink 8 ounces of water or sports drink
5:30–6:00 p.m.	A baked potato with nonfat sour cream or brown rice with steamed broccoli; an energy bar, if hungry Drink 8 ounces of water
7:00–7:30 p.m.	An energy bar Drink 8 ounces of water
9:00 p.m.	An energy bar, if hungry Drink 8 ounces of water

Marathon morning:

5:00 a.m.	Wake up Drink 8 ounces of water
6:00 a.m.	An energy bar and a cup of coffee Drink 8 ounces of water
6:30 a.m.	Drink 4 to 8 ounces of water, if there's no sloshing in the stomach
7:00 a.m.	Start race

Eating during the marathon

By eating blood-sugar-boosting snacks during long runs and the marathon, you can maintain your blood sugar level and stay more focused and motivated. Even when your legs are totally fatigued, your spirit can soar. The rule of thumb for the amount of blood sugar snacks consumed during long runs and marathons: 30–40 calories, every 2 miles, starting about mile 5.

The long runs serve as your testing ground for your stomach. I eat an energy bar (around 230 calories) before long runs and find that my BSL remains stable for 8 to 10 miles. About 60 to 90 minutes into a long run or marathon, start reloading with your snack of choice (always taken with water). If you didn't eat before the start, your blood-sugar boosters should begin at the 10- to 15-minute mark. It doesn't pay to wait until the level goes down to prop it up. The frequency and amount of gel or other snacks should be adjusted on long runs so that you know what to do on marathon day. If you are nauseous at the end of a long run, you probably ate too much at one time, didn't drink enough water, or overloaded the system with a sports drink. If your BSL drops at the end, you need to increase the amount or frequency of your booster snack all the way to the end of the run. It's usually better to eat smaller amounts more often.

If you're among the few runners who have digestive problems with even the smallest quantities of gel during a run, try hard candies or Gummi Bears. Of course, you don't want anything so large that you could choke on it. Sucking on one hard candy per mile (and drinking water) has not caused problems for anyone so far as I know.

WHAT TO AVOID

Salt

Salt consumed during the 24 hours before the marathon will raise the sodium concentration of the blood. Fluid is then taken from muscle tissue and other areas, causing dehydration and reducing your capacity for performance.

Fat

The more fat you eat the day before a long run (especially after 2 p.m.), the more sluggish your digestive system becomes and the less effective the food will be in delivering nutrients that can be used during the marathon. Because it takes a longer time to process, a fatty meal often causes stomach or bowel problems the next day.

Fiber

Too much loading up on fiber foods the day before can lead to unloading during the long run or on marathon morning. This is not only embarrassing, but also dehydrating.

Alcohol

A central nervous system depressant, alcohol will leave you with less motivation the next morning, thus interfering with your goal, whether it be for a time or to finish. Alcohol is also a major dehydrating agent.

Large meals

After a large meal the night before long runs or marathons, much of that food will still be in your intestines the following morning, drawing blood away from the exercising muscles. *Note:* Loading up on food the day before can cause unloading during the marathon.

VII PRACTICAL ADVICE

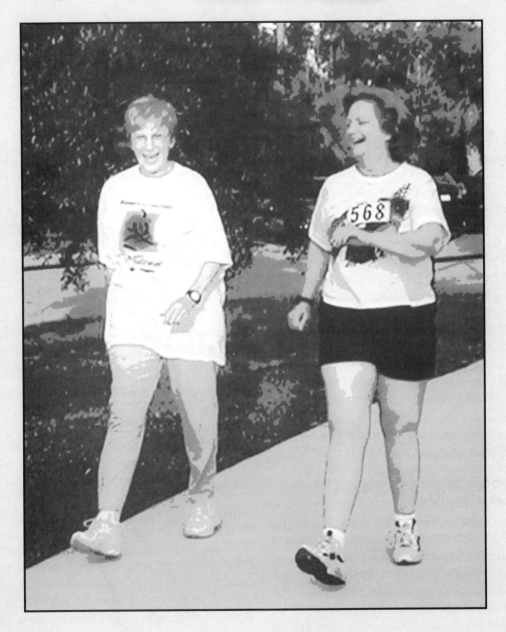

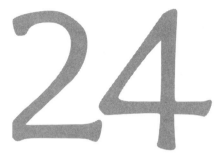

GETTING OLDER

"I feel better, at age 78, than I have felt in my 45 years of running. Slower, yes, but much happier with my running."

Recently, after a 10-mile race, I met a runner who was 93 years old. He was mentally alert and just as fired up about finishing as any of the other runners. The number of runners is growing, but the segment of those over 80 years of age is growing faster. These folks are clearly showing that the joys of running continue at any age.

Yes, the endorphins are the same at age 80 as they are at age 20. And the benefits of extra vitality and a positive attitude cannot be derived from any pills or any other activity I know. An 86-year-old man who ran 30 miles a week told me that his sedentary wife was constantly chiding him for not settling down and acting his age. He solved the problem when he started running during her regular naps. His mileage increased and she didn't know any better.

No bone or joint damage after 50 years of running!

Twenty-five years ago, many well-meaning doctors (who didn't run) told me that, if I continued to run, I could expect to be using a cane to walk by the time I reached the age of 55. I'm proud to say that I've passed that barrier and am now averaging more than 40 miles a week and enjoying every one of them.

I'm actually part of a study. In the early 1970s, Dr. David Costill, a physiologist, and Dr. Kenneth Cooper, the founder of the Aerobics Institute in Dallas, Texas, joined forces in a landmark study of world-class athletes. I was proud to be invited as a subject of this study. Over the past decade, we have been checked periodically to see how much we've deteriorated. After bone scans, CAT scans, and X-rays of all major joint areas, I received a clean bill of orthopedic health. *Note:* Studies show that runners have healthier joints than non-runners, even after more than 30 years of running.

How about arthritis? Two studies of runners have been done over 40- and 50-year periods. Both showed less incidence of arthritis and other joint problems for runners as opposed to non-runners. Other experts have told me that runners who are genetically predisposed to arthritis will get it but later in life and with less severe symptoms. A recent study showed that runners over 50 had 25% fewer orthopedic complaints compared with non-running peers.

If running could destroy joints and cartilage, mine would have been destroyed. During my competitive years, I pushed the edge, going over it into injury about every three weeks. I was so obsessed with performance that I continued to run, as hard as possible, until I could not. In dozens of cases, I had to take weeks or months off from running because I refused to take a day or two off at the first symptoms. Needless to say, I've had hundreds of injuries. Fortunately, our bodies are programmed to adapt to running and walking and they make adjustments. One X-ray specialist told me that I had the knees of a healthy 18-year-old. So now I want to pass on information about adjustments I've made that have not only made running more enjoyable but also kept me from having an overuse injury for more than fourteen years.

Vitality and attitude

If you're fit, age is not a factor. Sure, my muscles don't feel as good as they did even ten years ago—but that doesn't matter, as long as I check my ego at the door as I leave the house. It was a wonderful revelation that slowing down allows you to feel great—just about every day. The quality of my life has been based upon two factors: vitality and attitude. Running maintains both at the highest possible level. For most marathoners over the age of 50, attitude is often maintained at a lifetime best level. I believe that we become more introspective as we age. Running provides a positive outlet for this continuous inward journey and more time to oneself to organize the brain and get things on track.

For runners over the age of 50, fatigue is related to the number of running days per week and only indirectly to the number of miles per week. For example, many runners have felt better by taking an extra day

or two off per week, while maintaining the same weekly mileage. Our recovery rate slows down each year. By taking more days off from running, we speed up the rebuilding process. At the same time, a higher level of performance can often be achieved by increasing the number of miles run on a running day. Speed and endurance sessions that are specifically designed for the marathon, for example, have allowed many runners to improve as they have graduated to the next age group.

HOW MANY DAYS OFF PER WEEK?

Those who are having aches, extra fatigue, etc. can cut back the number of training days to the following:

- 40-year-old long distance runners and walkers need three days off from running.
- Over 50-year-old long distance runners and walkers should shift to every other day running or walking.
- Over-60 folks should run or walk three days per week and monitor for fatigue.
- The over-70 crowd can maintain a significant level of performance by training two days a week and taking an endurance walk or water running session as a third workout each week.

Performance tips for the over-40 crowd

The older you are, the longer it takes to recover from fatigue and injury. So, once you are over 40, getting better as you get older means that you need to make adjustments to your training schedule and to your running form.

Run more often

Run twice a day on the running days. Take the first run very slowly. If you want a little speed play, do some accelerations or hills on the second run—but be careful.

Accelerations

Accelerations maintain a high leg turnover. Keep your feet low to the ground—stride short. While staying light on your feet, pick up the rhythm after about 100 to 150 meters, and glide by reducing the effort while maintaining the turnover.

- Marathoners in their 50s can do accelerations on three of the afternoon runs.
- Marathoners in their 60s can do accelerations twice a week on the afternoon runs.
- Marathoners in their 70s can do accelerations once a week on an afternoon run.

Remember that accelerations are merely increased-turnover drills; they are not sprints. If your legs are tired or too tight, don't do the accelerations.

The long run pace

Run at a pace that is 3 minutes per mile slower than you could run that distance on that day. Yes, this is a minute slower than younger runners would go, but it will give you the same endurance, based upon the mileage covered. Remember to account for heat, humidity, hills, and other factors as you set your pace. I start my long runs about 4 minutes per mile slower than I could race the distance, and not only do I feel great at the end of the run, but also, in two days, I'm almost always recovered, even from a 26-miler. I know, I can see the looks on the faces of you competitive runners. Sure, it will take longer to complete these long runs, but this just gives you more time to brag about your grandchildren. In our marathon training groups, grandparents have a priceless opportunity: a captive audience for several hours!

Length

Increase the length of the long run beyond 26 miles. The only purpose of the long run is to build endurance. The slower you go, the quicker you'll recover. By having at least one long run beyond 26 miles, you can boost your endurance limit, which will allow you to maintain a hard marathon pace for a longer time in the marathon itself. When you go the extra distance, it is crucial to take the walk breaks and adhere to the pacing guidelines. For maximum performance, your longest run should be 28 to 29 miles. And, I'll say it again: you must go extra slowly on those extra-long runs.

Walk breaks

Take walk breaks every mile, from the beginning, to reduce fatigue. Put in a 1-minute walk break every 1–3 minutes of running from the beginning. Walk breaks do not reduce the endurance value of the run.

Schedule

Alternate long runs with other weekend runs. Until your long run reaches 18 miles, you may run it every other weekend. After that point, run long every third weekend. When the long run reaches 26 miles, you have the option of taking four weeks between long runs. On the other weekends, you may take a slow run of half the distance of your current long run or race a 5K —but nothing longer than 5K.

XT or cross training

While XT is not required for finishing, it will improve overall conditioning. On days between runs, a different form of exercise will slightly boost performance without pounding. Water running and cross-country ski machines produce the most direct improvement. Walking, rowing, and bicycling are great for recovery and bestow some indirect benefits. Swimming and weight training help to balance the muscle development of the body but don't improve your running. Stair machines, high-impact aerobics, and leg-strengthening exercises are not recommended and can slow down the recovery process. If you don't have time, you can eliminate the cross training.

Note: Research tells us that for every hour we exercise, we can statistically expect 2 hours extended to our life span.

Age magnifies the damage

Even young athletes will suffer if they make the following mistakes. Because recovery rate slows down each year, the damage caused by stepping over the line is more dramatic and long-lasting in those of us who are, shall we say, challenged by age. The best strategy is, as always, prevention.

Junk miles

Running even a few miles on a day when you should be resting prevents the muscles from recovering fully. You're better off not running at all on an easy day and adding those miles to a running day—either as part of an extra warm-up or warm-down or as an additional run.

Starting too fast

Whether on a slow training run or in a race, a pace that is too fast in the beginning will cause a slowdown at the end and/or damage to the muscles, requiring a longer recovery time. It is always better to start out at a slower pace than you think you can maintain. Over the age of 50 practically all personal best performances are accomplished by running the second half of a race faster than you ran the first.

Over-striding

When runners (of all ages) err with the length of their running stride, they tend to over-stride. The consequences, in terms of tendon and muscle damage and the recovery time required for healing, are worse if you're over 50. Runners are most likely to over-stride when tired at the end of long runs, races, or speed sessions. To avoid this problem, work on a lighter step with a shorter stride. It should feel like you are lowering tension in the hamstrings.

Over-stretching

Many runners mistakenly try to "stretch out" tension produced by fatigue in the running muscles. Massage is a better treatment. When you feel that you've overdone it, don't stretch the area for an extended period of time; talk to a therapist about massage, and ask your doctor if anti-inflammatory medication is okay.

Over-exertion

Young or old, every runner pushes too far when doing higher performance speed or hill sessions. Again, it is the older runners who have to pay dearly with longer down time. Be particularly careful when running faster than you have been running in the recent past.

Increase the number of speed or hill repetitions very gradually. By taking more rest between repetitions, you'll reduce the chance of overuse injury and speed up the recovery time after each session. When doing a repeat mile session, for example, 40-year-olds should take at least a 4-minute walk between repeats. 50-year-olds need at least a 5-minute walk; 60-year-olds, at least a 6-minute walk; and those over 70, a 7- to 10-minute walk between repeats (or run twice as many 800s with a 4- to 5-minute walk between them).

Big runners

Tall and heavy runners take more stress on every step and find it harder to run continuously. Carrying around extra weight is like adding 10 to 30 years to your age.

There's good news, however. By putting in more walk breaks, early and often, running becomes easier and much more fun. You'll recover much more quickly while enjoying the end of the run more than ever.

Note: For more information on age/running issues, see my book *Running Until You're 100* (www.JeffGalloway.com).

Age	Fitness Level	Pounds Overweight	Your legs feel like you are:
20–29	very fit	10–20	30–39
20–29	average	10–20	35–45
20–29	unfit	10–20	40–50
20–29	very fit	over 20	35–45
20–29	average	over 20	40–50
20–29	unfit	over 20	45–55
30–39	very fit	10–20	40–49
30–39	average	10–20	45–55
30–39	unfit	10–20	50–60
30–39	very fit	over 20	45–55
30–39	average	over 20	50–60
30–39	unfit	over 20	55–65
40–49	very fit	10–20	50–60
40–49	average	10–20	55–65
40–49	unfit	10–20	60–70
40–49	very fit	over 20	55–65
40–49	average	over 20	60–70
40–49	unfit	over 20	65–75
50–59	very fit	10–20	60–69
50–59	average	10–20	65–75
50–59	unfit	10–20	70–80
50–59	very fit	over 20	65–75
50–59	average	over 20	70–80
50–59	unfit	over 20	75–85

MY FAVORITE MARATHON COMPANION

Before I started running, I had been a fat and inactive kid. Like many boys, I wanted to be like my Dad. In the eighth grade, I tried the sport in which he had achieved "all-state" status: football. At first I sensed that my temperament (and weight) wasn't quite right for the sport ("Hit 'em harder, Galloway! Make 'em feel your impact!"). By the end of that season, I *knew* that the sport that was supposed to "make a man of you" wasn't for me.

My dad steered me into cross-country running, where I felt instantly at home. I'm only guessing, but any parent would tend to want his or her child to hang out with the type of kids that run distance events. Then, as today, these athletes tend to be better students and leaders. I found them to be interesting and fun to run with. When my progress seemed to stagnate, my dad brought me some reading material about various training programs, including those of the great New Zealand coach Arthur Lydiard. These readings gave me the principles that I use to this day.

As I moved on to college, I became fitter as my sedentary Dad became fatter. By my mid-twenties, continuing to read about fitness, I became concerned about my father's health as he tipped the scales above 200 pounds. Not aware of the way our health is influenced by such factors, he complained about aches and pains and displayed an increasingly negative attitude. He read the book *Aerobics*, but his sedentary behavior didn't change. On one occasion, when I suggested walking around the park in front of his office, he explained that his varicose veins and allergies prevented him from exercising. I stopped arguing with him.

When he was fifty-two, a high school reunion changed his life. At this gathering of the Moultrie, Georgia, class of '37, he discovered that, of twenty-five boys in that class who had been on the football team, thirteen had died of degenerative diseases. Of all the activities of the weekend, this fact weighed on his mind on the three-and-a-half hour drive back home. By the time he turned into his driveway, Elliott Galloway realized that he could be the next one to drop from the roster, and he decided to do something about it.

Starting at a particular telephone pole, he set off that first day, determined to run the three-mile loop across the street from his office. Reality was harsh. He had to settle for only the next telephone pole, about 100 meters away. On each successive run, the goal was one additional pole, until he made it completely around. Almost two years later he was running 10K races. Seven years later, and 55 pounds lighter, he was running marathons, including one below the three-hour mark.

Having had an irregular heart rhythm for years, he decided, upon receiving doctor's orders, to finish his marathon career in 1996 at the one hundredth running of the Boston Marathon. He consented to let me tag along with him. It would be my one hundredth marathon finish and the one I will remember for the rest of my life most vividly.

As we started, the thought hit me that the Boston Marathon had only been run twenty-three times when my Dad was born. As best I could, I forced him to walk at each mile mark. (You see, he doesn't listen to what I say!) I had run Boston four other times, pushing as hard as I could each time. As we shared our enjoyment of the scenery, the energetic crowd, and the landmarks, it all seemed new to me. Oxygen debt must blank out your memory cells. This was a day for savoring, and we did just that.

As we turned the corner and saw the finish structure, my Dad took off. We were zooming down the final straight as the clock ticked away toward a time barrier that we were determined to break: six hours. We did: 5:59:48. He told anyone who asked about the race that he would have run much faster if I hadn't slowed him down.

I never disagreed.

25 INJURIES & INTERRUPTIONS

For runners, the most common sites of injury are the knee, the foot, the Achilles tendon, and the ankle: weak links that are the most susceptible. By taking a day or two off from running, at the first sign of an injury, you can avoid two to three weeks, or months of down time later.

Everyone has a weak link. Each of us, because of our individual biomechanics and structured patterns of motion, tend to aggravate specific areas of our bodies over and over. When we exercise too many days per week or increase the intensity or mileage too rapidly, these sites are usually the first to react. This effect can be very useful, giving us an early warning signal to back off before we push into injury. Marathon training is more likely to reveal the weak links than other forms of exercise.

BE AWARE OF AREAS THAT:

- Get sore first, or swell up
- Are repeatedly sore, painful, or inflamed
- Take longer to warm up
- Have been injured before
- Are not functioning in their usual way

As you become more sensitive to such areas, you'll take time off for recovery and treatment at the earliest of warning signs. Quick and early action will cut down on the chance that you'll have to spend weeks or months of recovery later.

Signs of injury

- **Inflammation:** Look for swelling around the injury site.
- **Loss of function:** The muscle, foot, tendon, and so on doesn't work the way it should.
- **Pain** that increases or lasts consistently for a week or more.

Inflammation

Inflammation is the body's attempt to immobilize an injured area to keep you from damaging it further. The excess fluid around the injury notifies you that there is a problem. Your range of motion is reduced and this normally limits the extent of further damage. External swelling, such as the swollen area around a sprained ankle, is usually apparent.

Internal inflammation is harder to spot. At joints, tendon connections, and in small areas of muscle, it takes only a little bit of inner swelling to reduce the capacity of the muscle and produce pain. Be very sensitive to the possible minor muscle or tendon pulls or strains in areas such as behind the knee, at the intersection between hamstring and butt muscle, the adductors, the abductors, and the lower back muscles.

Many runners have reported that anti-inflammatory medications (such as ibuprofen) taken immediately after a difficult run can significantly reduce the chance of inflammation and injury and speed healing. Be sure to talk to your doctor before taking even over-the-counter medications because all have some side effects. Taking any medication before or during a long run (or the marathon) is not recommended. Whenever taking medications, follow the advice of your doctor and the instructions on the container, and discontinue their use at the first sign of potential problems.

Loss of function

If the tendon, muscle, or other injured part is not doing its job, don't ignore it. By continuing to run, you're very likely to injure it further. Running with an injury can produce a new injury. When a muscle, tendon, and so on doesn't function to capacity, the workload of running shifts to other components that are not designed to handle the stress. In many cases, this causes a series of compensation injuries.

Pain that doesn't go away

Temporary aches and pains will come and go throughout a marathon program, usually disappearing after a day or so, and thus indicating that you probably don't have an injury. But if the pain increases or continues for five to seven days, treat it as an injury: Take at least two days off from running and use ice and other treatments as necessary. Continuing pain, even without loss of function, can be an early sign of internal inflammation.

Don't stretch tight muscles

It's a mistake to stretch a muscle to its limits when it feels tight or fatigued. Stretching can actually cause injuries if done the wrong way (bouncing, or pushing too far). If your running muscles are tight from exercise try massage, walking, or a shortening of stride length before stretching.

The fatigue of long runs and speed sessions will tighten the muscles and reduce strength and range of motion. Stretching fatigued muscles can tear the fatigued fibers, producing injury and increasing recovery time. If you over-stretch a tired muscle, you engage the stretch reflex. This protective mechanism tightens the muscle in order to protect it. Take care in stretching at the end of long runs or speed sessions, since fatigue will loosen the connections, and you may stretch the muscles into an overextended position. When in doubt, don't stretch.

Injuries: how to treat them

Consult a doctor

Choose a doctor or health professional who knows running. Getting a good diagnosis can speed the treatment and get you back on the roads quicker. A good doctor's advice and treatment can speed recovery by several weeks. It can often mean the difference between whether you will make it to the starting line of your marathon or not.

Don't stretch an injured muscle

Until it heals, an injured area should not be stretched—unless you've injured the *iliotibial* band, in which case, ask your doctor what measures are appropriate.

Stop using the injured part

For at least two to five days refrain from using the injured part. In most cases your doctor will tell you that the injury doesn't have to heal completely before you run again; but you must get the healing started and continue a program that doesn't cause injury. Again, talk to the Doc. When in doubt, stay below the threshold of further irritation.

Ice

If the injury site is near the surface of the body, ice massage usually helps. Be sure to use a chunk of ice (made by putting paper or styrofoam cups of water in the freezer) and rub it directly on the injured area until it is numb (usually about 10 to 15 minutes). This is particularly helpful for all tendon and other foot injuries. Be sure to ice at the first sign of injury, ice as soon as possible after exercise, and keep icing for at least a week after the pain goes away. The regularity of the ice treatment is very important so do it every day! In deeper tendon or muscle injuries, ice treatment may not have any effect but should cause no harm.

Note: Do not ice for over 15 minutes; you don't want to *freeze* the area.

Compression

Compression will help to restrain further inflammation. Wrapping a sprained ankle soon after injury will reduce the inflammation. This is another remedy for which you should get advice from your running-oriented physician.

Note: You must release compression regularly.

Elevation

To reduce inflammation, an injured leg, for example, would be elevated on a pillow or two as you read or watch TV in bed.

Massage

To speed up the healing of muscle injuries dramatically, massage is often helpful. A massage therapist or physical therapist who is experienced in working with runners should be able to advise you whether your injury will heal quicker with massage and when it's time to work on it. Immediately after injury is not usually a good time.

Getting back to running

Do you have to start all over if your marathon program is interrupted? Probably not. Most of us are not in a position to quit our job and leave our family and other responsibilities to train for a marathon and so must steer our aerobic ship around the obstructions. There are as many ways to rebuild from a layoff as there are problems that cause the interruptions.

Note: Water running and long walks can maintain most of your running adaptations (if the injury allows).

Injury timetable

- At the first sign of an injury, or even an aggravated weak link, take an extra day or two off.

- If it's an injury, see a doctor and get treatment immediately; the sooner treated, the sooner healed.

- Immediately start a different type of exercise, one that will not compound the injury; the sooner started, the more fitness retained.

- Make sure the healing is continuing as you ease gently back into running.
- Stay in touch with your doctor or physical therapist to limit the risk of re-injury.
- Continue to treat the injury as prescribed by the doctor. Ice massage, for example, should be continued every day for two weeks after the disappearance of all symptoms.

For more information on injuries, see *Galloway's Book on Running*.

After sickness

- If Doc allows you to do some low-level exercise, say 30 minutes, three times a week, do it!
- Always avoid the chance of lowering resistance to disease and getting sick again.
- Return to running conservatively.

Interruptions

Brief interruptions

For interruptions (sickness, injury, etc.) of less than 14 days, because of business, travel, vacation, and so on, you can work up to your normal weekly mileage in about the same number of days you took off from running.

- But every run must be done slowly: follow the Two-Minute Rule.
- You may increase the length of your run in a shorter time but only if you slow down your running pace and take more walk breaks on every run.
- It's always better to run every other day as you come back.

Longer interruptions

The longer your layoff from exercise, the more conservative your comeback must be. To determine the distance of your first long run after an extended layoff, first decide when you plan to begin your long runs again. Then, count back three weeks from that date. Use, as a starting point, the longest distance you were running before you interrupted the training. Then:

- Take off 20 percent per week if you have done no exercise at all in the meantime.
- Take off 10 percent per week if you did 30 minutes of alternative exercise, three times a week.
- Take off 5 percent per week if you did alternative exercise that simulated the marathon schedule.

For example, Chris ran 23 miles five weeks ago. Three days after that, he ran too hard on the mile repeats and injured his Achilles tendon. He did no running for three weeks, then he ran easy every other day for ten days. In addition, he had either run in the water or exerted himself on a cross-country ski machine about every other day, but only for short periods of time.

Now, about four and a half weeks later, his Achilles tendon felt secure enough for a long run. In choosing a distance for his first long run, he would have the following options:

- A 4- to 5-mile long run, if he had done no exercise at all during the layoff
- A 10- to 13-mile run if he had done 30 minutes of exercise three times a week
- A 23-mile run if he had been doing alternative exercise that simulated his marathon schedule, especially a long walk or water run every 2–3 weeks, comparable to about 20 miles

He decided that 15 miles would be his target for his first long run after the injury, and had no trouble resuming his marathon training.

Pacing the long run after a break

The first 2 miles should be run 3 to 4 minutes per mile more slowly than you could run that distance. Then, you can settle into a pace that is 3 minutes per mile slower or maintain your original pace. Take walk breaks twice as often.

Before his injury, Chris was taking a 1-minute break for every 4 minutes of running. When he started his comeback, he took a 1-minute break every 2 minutes. A runner who usually runs for 3 minutes and walks for 1 minute would, in starting back in again, run for 1 minute and walk for 1 minute, or 30 seconds/30seconds.

Increasing the distance

Be careful about pushing your body to get yourself back into marathon range.

- When you are running more than 3 minutes per mile slower than you could run and taking walk breaks twice as long and twice as frequently as you did before the interruption, you can increase the distance by no more than 4 to 5 miles per run.

- When you are running 2 to 3 minutes per mile slower than you could run and taking walk breaks twice as frequently as you were before the interruption, you can increase the distance by no more than 3 miles per run.

- When you are running 2 minutes per mile slower than you could run and taking walk breaks as frequently as you were before the interruption, increase the distance by no more than 2 miles per run.

"Somebody once told me that the difference between Olympians and the rest of the athletic community is that Olympians don't get injured, so they can keep training and making progress when others are stalled out by injuries. I think that's true, and for once, thanks to Jeff's approach to running I'm training as if I were an Olympian. Forward progress with no backtracking."

26 BREATHING

BREATHING

By using an efficient breathing technique, you'll not only be capable of a higher level of performance in the marathon but also you'll teach yourself how to acquire a better supply of oxygen and improve almost every aspect of your exercise experience. You'll also feel better doing the other things you do. In deep breathing (also called "belly breathing"), you're filling up the lower part of the lungs first. Through practice you can quickly inhale and quickly exhale while deep breathing and you don't need to fill the upper part of your lungs to capacity.

Deep-breathing technique

- Every third or fourth breath, quickly exhale as completely as possible.

- This almost guarantees a complete lower lung intake as you inhale immediately afterward.

- Breathe normally in between the deeper breaths.

- Don't do this deeper breathing more often because you could hyperventilate.

- You must start this technique from the beginning of your run to maximize its effect.

Some folks time their exhalations to take place as they push off for every second or third step. If this sounds interesting, try it two ways: (1) breathe out completely as you push off either the right or the left foot, or (2) alternate between the left or right foot. Compare the two methods, but it's better to try only one method during any specific run.

You can practice this breathing method at any time—not just when exercising. Be sure to start each exercise session using this technique. After several weeks or months of regular breathing in this way, it will become almost automatic.

Eliminating side pains

The deep-breathing technique can help reduce or eliminate those irritating side pains that often erupt just when you're getting into your exercise. Such pains seem to be caused primarily by shallow breathing—using the upper part of our lungs in a minimal way. This low-energy method of expenditure is adequate for our normal sedentary activities and seems to provide sufficient oxygen at the beginning of an exercise session. But it also limits the amount of oxygen that you can absorb during exertion and often puts you into debt. If you start your runs with shallow breathing, you'll probably get side pains during some of them. Side pains are aggravated if you go out faster than you should (even when the pace feels easy), so slow down at the beginning of all of your runs if you've been having this problem.

For more information on breathing, see *Galloway's Book on Running.*

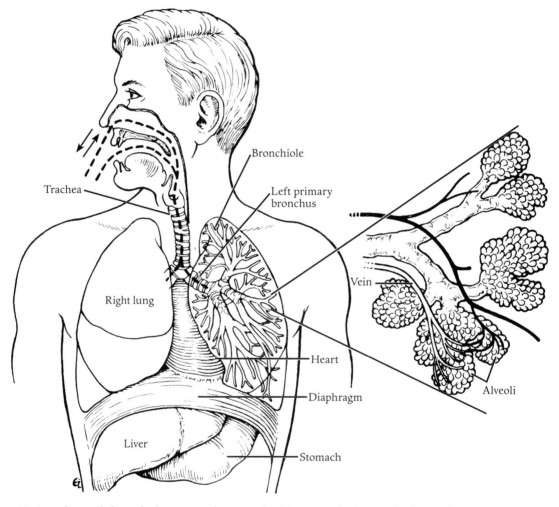

Air is exchanged through the nose and/or mouth. Air enters the lungs via the trachea, which branches to form the bronchi, which in turn branch, tree-like, to form smaller subdivisions, the bronchioles. Here a terminal bronchiole is enlarged to illustrate the air sacs (alveoli), in which exchange of gases takes place between air and blood.

27 RUNNING HOT AND COLD

COLD WEATHER RUNNING

Experts in extreme temperature research tell me that, even when the temperature drops to minus 30 degrees F (without the wind), there's no reason to be concerned about lung damage. There are numerous buffer zones in your respiratory system that prevent outside air from affecting any area deeper than your mouth, and masks can prevent problems there. By putting on the right combination of layers, fabrics, extremity protectors, and skin-care products, you can enjoy running on very cold days, as do the runners in Alaska, Minnesota, and the ice belt of Canada.

Dressing

Don't be held hostage by the weather. Visit a good running or ski store and find the right clothing. Wear a series of thin layers.

- Close to your skin, you'll want something warm. Polypropelene is one of several fibers that keep the warmth close to the skin, but allow extra heat and perspiration to escape. (Mizuno has a fiber that warms you as you perspire.)
- Add external layers, adjusting to the temperature and wind conditions.
- Cover up all extremities — hands, ears, toes — with extra layering.

- Men should wear an extra layer or two as underwear if necessary.
- In extreme cold (when the temperature or wind chill factor is below 10 degrees F [minus 11 degrees Centigrade]), do not expose any skin, if possible. Even when there is minimal exposure, put Vaseline or other cold weather insulation and protection on any area that may incidentally be hit by the wind, such as your eyelids, etc.
- Be sure to coat your shoes or use socks that insulate your feet. Most running shoes are designed to let heat out and cold into your feet. This can cause frostbite on days colder than 32 degrees F (or 0 degrees C). Remember that running itself can generate a significant wind chill effect on your feet. As you warm up while running, peel off each layer before you start sweating. Too much sweat accumulating will freeze and cause problems.

Warm-ups in winter

On very cold days, bundle up and exercise for a very few minutes indoors. You may walk, jog in place, use an indoor track, or exercise on the machines (cycle, rowing, stairs). Before you start sweating, go outdoors and you'll have a reservoir of warmth to get you down the road. Start your run or walk by going into the wind. This allows you to come back with the wind.

If you start to get very warm, remove an outside layer of clothing or unzip your outer layer. A garment with long sleeves may be tied around your waist, or put it in your fanny pack—you may need it later.

On cold days, pick environments where you could seek refuge for at least a few minutes if you need to. On very cold or windy days, alternate between inside and out. If you have an indoors facility, it helps to come inside when you start to get cold. Exercise indoors only long enough to take the sting away—but head outdoors before you start sweating.

CLOTHING THERMOMETER

These are recommendations only; use the combination of layers that works best for you.

Degrees F	What to wear as it gets colder
60 +	Tank top or singlet and shorts
50–59	T-shirt and shorts
40–49	Long-sleeved T-shirt, shorts or tights or wind pants, mittens or gloves
30–39	Long-sleeve T-shirt and another T-shirt, tights and shorts, socks, mittens or gloves, and a hat over your ears
20–29	Polypro top or thick long-sleeved T-shirt, another T-shirt layer, tights and shorts, socks, mittens or gloves, and a hat over your ears
10–19	Polypro top and thick long-sleeved T-shirt, tights and shorts, wind suit (top and pants), socks, thick mittens, and a thick hat over your ears
0–9	Two polypro tops, thick tights and shorts (and thick underwear or supporter for men), warm-up suit of Gore-Tex or a similar fabric, gloves and thick mittens, ski mask, a hat over your ears, and Vaseline covering any exposed skin
Minus 15–19	Two thick polypro tops, tights and thick polypro tights, thick underwear (and supporter for men), thick warm-up suit, gloves, thick (arctic) ski mask and a thick hat over your ears, Vaseline covering any exposed skin, thicker socks on your feet and other foot protection, as needed
Minus 20 and below	Add layers as needed

Stay in touch with the outdoor and ski shops for the warmest clothing that is still thin. Watch your feet. There are socks that may be heated up, not to mention other innovations.

HOT WEATHER RUNNING

There's good and bad news about running in the heat. First, the bad news: When the temperature rises above 55 degrees F (10 degrees C), you're going to run more slowly and feel worse than you will at lower temperatures. But by gradually preparing yourself for increased temperatures and taking action from the beginning of hot weather runs, you'll get a welcome dose of the good news. You'll learn how to hydrate yourself, what to wear, and when and how much your body can take in hot weather, all of which will help you recover faster and run better than others of your ability on hot days. While even the most heat-adapted runners won't run as fast on hot days as they can on cold ones, they won't slow down as much nor will they feel as much discomfort.

Note: Be sure to read the next section, Heat Disease Alert *(p. 174)*. Without knowing these concepts, you can get into serious trouble even on moderately warm days. Mark that section and revisit it several times during the warm season of the year. If you have any risk of heart disease, talk to a doctor trained in exercise before continuing.

Until the temperature rises to about 65 degrees F, most runners don't notice much heat buildup, even though it is already putting extra burdens on the system. It takes most folks about 30 to 45 minutes of running (with or without walk breaks) to feel warm. But soon after that, if the temperature is above about 62 degrees F, you're suddenly hot and sweating. On runs and especially races under those conditions, most runners have to force themselves to slow down. It's just too easy to start faster than you should when the temperature is between 60 and 69 degrees F because it feels cool at first.

As the mercury rises above 65 degrees F, your body can't get rid of the heat building up. This causes a rise in core body temperature and an early depletion of fluids through sweating. The internal temperature rise also triggers the rapid dispersion of blood into the capillaries of the skin, reducing the amount of that vital fluid that is available to the exercising muscles. Just when those workhorses are being pushed to capacity, they are receiving less oxygen and nutrients. What used to be a river becomes a creek and can't remove the waste products of exercise (such as lactic acid). As these accumulate, your muscles slow down.

Note: I've found that runners slow down 30 seconds per mile with every 5-degree temperature increase above 60°F. If you make this adjustment, you should avoid heat stress and pass a lot of runners at the end.

Body fat

The more body fat you have, the worse you'll feel as the temperature and humidity rise. I don't have any research on this, but my experience tells me that for every increase of 5 percent in body fat, the effects of heat and humidity are felt about 5 minutes sooner. For example, if a runner with 12 percent body fat feels severe heat discomfort after 45 minutes of running, then a runner with 22 percent body fat will feel it after 35 minutes, and a runner with 32 percent body fat after 25 minutes. Body fat acts like a blanket to hold heat in. It does too good a job during the summer.

Scheduling

The best time for hot weather running is before sunrise. The more you can run before sunrise, the cooler you will feel, compared with how you'll feel later in the day. The second best time to run, by the way, is right after sunrise, unless the temperature cools off dramatically at sunset, which would make that time more favorable. In humid areas, however, it usually doesn't cool down much after sunset.

How to stay cool at 55 degrees F or above

Slow down early: 30 seconds per mile for every 5°F above 60°F

The later you wait to slow down, the more dramatically you'll slow down at the end and the longer it will take to recover from the run. Walk breaks, early and often, help you lower the exertion level, which conserves resources for the end and reduces heat buildup.

Wear lighter garments

Loose-fitting clothes allow heat to escape. Don't wear cotton clothing. Sweat soaks into cotton, causing it to cling to your skin, increasing heat buildup. Several materials will wick the perspiration away from your skin: Coolmax, polypro, etc. As moisture leaves your skin, you receive a cooling effect, and these types of materials are designed for this.

Pour water over yourself

Up to 70 percent of the heat you can lose goes out through the top of your head so regularly pour water over your hair (even if, like me, you are hair challenged). Regularly pouring water on a light, polypro (or a similar material) singlet or tank top will keep you cooler.

Don't wear a hat

Hats keep the heat from being released through the best vent you have, the top of your head. Don't cover it up.

Drink cold water

Not only does cold water leave the stomach of a runner quicker than any type of fluid, it produces a slight physiological cooling effect—and an even greater psychological cooling effect. But don't drink too much either. Most of us do well with between 6 and 10 ounces an hour during warm weather. Drink until you hear sloshing in your stomach, then stop. When the sloshing sound goes away, resume drinking.

Take a dip or a shower

On hot days, you can reduce heat buildup significantly if you spend 3 or 4 minutes in a pool or cold shower every mile or two. Do this several times and even the hottest day's run becomes manageable. The break in your run will not cause you to get out of shape. Over the span of a month, most runners get in more training this way because they don't overheat early.

Don't eat a big meal

Eating too much, particularly meals that are high in protein or fat, will put extra stress on your system when you exercise. Even worse is the probability that too much food loading will lead to unloading during the run. That can be embarrassing! Instead of big meals, eat light, easily digestible snacks, every hour or two. Many runners find it better not to eat anything within two hours or so of their hot weather run (although energy bars or PowerGel work well for most, when taken 1–2 hours before the run).

Training for hot weather

One day a week, you can train yourself to deal with the heat by inserting the hot segments below into your run, even if you are starting in the middle of winter. Of course, you need to run at least two other days per week, and you must do this heat training day every week. Before running each hot segment, read p. 174 on symptoms of heat disease. At the first indication of symptoms, stop running before you get into trouble.

The process of heat training follows the same principles as conditioning for endurance and speed. By pushing yourself a little bit and then backing off, your body makes adaptations and can deal with the heat better the next time. On each run, warm up for at least 10 minutes of easy running (and walking), and ease off with at least 10 minutes of easy running (and walking) after the heat phase. If the outdoor temperature is cool, you may put on one or more layers of clothes, especially on the upper body, during the hot segment. You may also do these segments indoors. Take it very easy on these segments. You're only working on heat adaptation, not speed or intensity.

Schedule of Hot Segments

Week Number	Duration of Hot Segment
1	5–7 minutes
2	7–9 minutes
3	9–12 minutes
4	12–16 minutes
5	16–22 minutes
6	22–26 minutes

Adjusting for heat

As the weather gets hotter, you must slow down your pace from the beginning. Also, in most places in North America, you'll need to make adjustments for the humidity. The higher the humidity, the sooner you'll feel the effect of the heat and the more difficult it will be to continue. Watch the weather reports and install a temperature and humidity gauge at your house. After a while, you'll learn the combination of the two that causes you discomfort and can avoid the times of the day when those conditions arise.

TALLAHASSEE SHOWERS

In Tallahassee, I discovered an outdoor shower beside the FSU track. Practically every afternoon during June, July, and August, I'd structure my runs so that I looped by the track at least every two miles. If my body heat built up more quickly, I'd cut the loop short and head for the shower. For those runs, I used special shoes that could be slipped on and off quickly without being unlaced. Without those regular dousings, I wouldn't have run half the distance I was able to cover.

HEAT DISEASE ALERT

Heat disease is a common health problem among endurance exercisers. This is a serious condition that has frequently resulted in death, even among highly trained, young athletes.

Symptoms

- Intense heat buildup in the head, significant headache, general overheating of the body
- General confusion and loss of concentration and muscular control
- Excessive sweating and then the cessation of sweating, a clammy skin, and excessively heavy breathing
- Extreme tiredness, upset stomach, muscle cramps, vomiting, and faintness

Risk factors

- Sleep deprivation
- Viral or bacterial infection
- Dehydration (avoid alcohol and caffeine)
- Severe sunburn and skin irritation
- Lack of acclimation to hot weather
- Overweight
- Lack of training for a specific training exercise
- Occurrence(s) of heat disease in the past
- Medications, especially cold medicines, diuretics, medicines for diarrhea, tranquilizers, antihistamines, atropine, and scopolamine
- Certain medical conditions including high cholesterol levels, high blood pressure, extreme stress, asthma, diabetes, epilepsy, drug use (including alcohol), cardiovascular disease, smoking, or a general lack of fitness

Prevention

- During hot weather, exercise at the coolest time (usually before sunrise).
- Drink water all day long, 4–8 oz. per hour when needed.
- Avoid caffeine, alcohol, and other drugs.
- Wear clothing that is light and loose.
- Eat small, lowfat snacks that you know will not cause you distress.
- Don't increase the duration or intensity of your exercise significantly.
- Slow down your pace even more to account for heat, humidity, and hills —especially in the beginning.
- Take walk breaks more often.

- See a physician who specializes in running and fitness before beginning the program if you have any questions about any of the conditions mentioned, or if you notice any significant change in body functions, immune response, and so on.

Take action!

Watch for heat disease in group members and take action if you think anyone is in trouble. Walk, cool off, and get help immediately.

HYPONATREMIA, OR WATER INTOXICATION:

Don't drink more than 20 oz/hour

While extremely rare, this condition has caused death during or after long runs or marathons. Many runners become overly concerned about hyponatremia, and don't drink enough before, during and after a long run. The result is dehydration, which is much more likely to cause medical problems, and increase recovery time after long runs. As in all training components, use good common sense.

The underlying cause of hyponatremia is often severe dehydration, compounded by consuming fluid in great quantities. Every marathoner should be aware of this condition, not only for self-protection. If you see someone who seems to be going through the symptoms, a little attention can bring them around relatively quickly. If a member of your running group shows any of the symptoms below, stay in touch with that person for the next few hours to ensure that he or she is getting what is needed and is not alone. As always, when in doubt, get medical advice and care. A physician will have to determine whether an IV will help or not.

Causes:

- Sweating excessively and continuously for more than 5 hours
- *and/or*
- Taking medication (within 48 hours of a long run) which messes up the fluid storage, and fluid balance systems
- *and*
- Drinking too much water

Signs that you may have it

- Hands and/or feet swell up twice normal size (or more)
- Nausea that leads to vomiting, continuous or several times
- Diarrhea which is continuous or repeated every 10 minutes or so
- Mental disorientation and confusion
- Severe cramping of the muscles for several miles

How to avoid it

1. Drink water in small doses during a long run—6–8 oz., no more often than every 25 minutes.
2. Don't drink if you hear a sloshing sound in your stomach.
3. After 2–3 hours of continuous, excessive sweating, eat salty pretzels, or mix a small packet of salt with your water, every 30 minutes or so.
4. Continue to eat or drink the salty food for an hour after a run of 5 hours or longer.
5. Drink a sip or so of water or electrolyte drink with every pretzel.
6. At the end of long runs, and for hours afterward, even if you are very thirsty, don't drink more than 8 oz. of water about every 30 minutes. It is OK to drink some electrolyte beverage which is not diluted.
7. The electrolyte beverages don't have enough sodium to get you back to balance, but the carbohydrate in them will slow down the absorption of the water.

Note: Strive to drink 2–4 ounces every 1–2 miles, but no more than 20 oz/hour.

28 HEART RATE MONITORS

A merry heart goes all day.
–Shakespeare, *The Winter's Tale*

Your heart rate is an excellent indicator of the intensity of your exercise, provided that you don't dramatically extend the length of the workout beyond the level to which you're currently trained. When you're running below 70 percent of your maximum heart rate, you are unlikely to over-train in intensity. (You can still over-train by going farther than you've trained to go.) By keeping the heart rate between 70 and 80 percent of your maximum rate, you can assume that your effort will normally produce a creative stress on the system, causing it to improve. This is the range you want to see during most of your speed workouts. But even the time spent in this 70- to 80-percent range must be managed so that you increase only gradually.

But, when you push the effort beyond 80 percent of your maximum heart rate, you increase the recovery time for that workout. For those looking for top performance, incursions into the 80-percent range and even the occasional 90-percent bout are fine (provided your doctor approves). Because your recovery time and risk of injury increase with the amount of time spent above 80 percent, the heart monitor can act as a damage-control device.

Hard workouts should be done only once a week, and you should ease into them. At first, make sure that you're spending only a few seconds at a time in the over-80-percent range. As the workouts progress, you can increase the length of the time over 80 percent a little and also increase the frequency. Monitor your increase: Track the total number of minutes spent above 70 percent, above 80 percent, and above 90 percent in each speed workout, and don't let the increase in any segment of any one workout exceed 25 percent of that of the week before.

Remember that overwork can be cumulative. Too many days per month of racing, speedwork, and long runs that are too fast can add up.

Before using a heart rate monitor, you must be tested by a trained professional to ascertain your maximum heart rate. You don't need to go through a maximum oxygen uptake test; the maximum heart rate test is sufficient and not as involved. Tables or formulas based on age are available, but are only averages. Before you monitor heart rate on long runs, however, read the long-run segment on p. 177.

Testing is important because, if you estimate your maximum heart rate and your guess is too low, you'll not receive as much benefit as you might from using the heart monitor on speed sessions and will be wasting one of the primary sources of biofeedback that the heart monitor can give. If your guess is too high, you'll over-train on speed sessions and risk a long recovery time. It's also possible to over-train on easy days and thus not recover between the harder sessions.

Heart monitors can help

- To hold you back during a long run —especially at the end
- To make sure that an easy day really is *easy*
- To ensure that form accelerations are easy gliders
- To improve your marathon racing form without over-training
- To keep you from needing a long recovery after marathon speed sessions
- To tell you when you have rested enough between mile repeats in a speed session
- To serve notice when you're over-trained and need to take some extra days off or to take things easy
- To make sure that you're not becoming increasingly tired on marathon-pace runs

Heart monitors don't help

- At the beginning of long runs, especially if you try to stay close to 70 percent of your maximum heart rate. (Use the Two-Minute Rule for pacing.)
- When you don't know your exact maximum heart rate. (Get tested, under supervision.)

Resting heart rate

Pick a time of the day when you're less likely to be influenced by psychological or emotional considerations that would influence your heart rate. For example, many find that the time right after waking is ideal. Each day, put on your monitor at this time and note your heart rate over a 5- to 10-minute time frame. If you have less time, shorten the test period. After a few weeks, you'll establish a base line that tells you your average heart rate. Over the span of 6 to 12 months, you will learn what the level is when you're rested, when you're training moderately hard, and when you're over-training.

When your resting heart rate (taken under the same conditions, day after day) is 5 percent higher than the low baseline, take an easy day. When the rate climbs to 10 percent or more higher than your low baseline, take the day off from running. You may do some non-pounding exercise if desired.

Controlling the pace

Almost everyone is capable of running faster for 3 to 6 miles than they can run for 15 miles or more. If you wear your heart monitor on a long training run and try to stay close to 70 percent of your maximum heart rate, you'll almost certainly run too hard at first, which will make the end of the run difficult and increase your recovery time.

Pacing the long run

At the start of a long run, you can run more slowly than you could race a 5K or 10K distance and feel very comfortable for the first few miles. But running at close to 70 percent of your maximum heart rate means that you're running at 70 percent of your 5K or 10K pace, which is almost certainly too fast for a run that will exceed 15 miles. In other words, you can run too fast during the first part of a long run, feel good, and still register a heart rate of less than 70 percent of maximum heart rate.

Use the Two-Minute Rule instead of your heart monitor during the first part of the long run and adjust your pace for heat, humidity, hills, and so on. Even if your pace is slower than this, you'll benefit with a faster recovery and still get the same endurance conditioning as you would from a fast run over the same distance.

The heart monitor can help you regulate subconscious increases in effort between pace checks. I recommend staying below 65 percent of your maximum heart rate for the first half of the long run. You'll probably notice an elevated rate on the hills (telling you to slow down). During the second half, the gradual onset of fatigue will cause the heart rate to rise naturally at the same effort level. Adjust your pace to keep the rate below 70 percent during the second half.

Pacing the easy runs

The easy runs during the week merely maintain the conditioning you gained on the weekend long run (or on the mile repeats). To ensure that you're running slowly enough, wear your heart monitor, and stay below 65 percent of your maximum. This conservative plan will prevent you from going too hard when you need to be recovering.

Monitoring for runners with time goals

It's beneficial for time-goal marathoners, if they have recovered from the weekend long or hard runs, to run at marathon pace on the easy runs during the week. Here are some guidelines for using a heart monitor while running parts of the easy-day runs at goal pace:

1. Run a slow warm-up, ensuring that your heart rate is significantly below 70 percent of maximum. If there are any signs of tiredness, run slowly for the rest of the session.

2. After 1 to 2 slow miles, do four to eight acceleration gliders. These will help your running form to become smoother while you become comfortable running at a faster rhythm.

3. As you start the first mile at marathon pace, monitor your heart rate. Ideally, the rate will stay around 70 percent of maximum, but it's okay if it creeps a bit higher. But, if the rate reaches 75 percent of maximum and you're not running faster than goal pace, it's a sign that you're still fatigued from earlier sessions; run slowly for the rest of the session.

Accelerations, not sprints

The purpose of gliding fast during some of your easy weekday runs is to work on more efficient form. You want these quicker-turnover glides of 100 meters or so to be at a faster pace than you would run normally but without requiring a significant increase in effort or heart rate. The heart monitor can give you this check on reality. If the rate rises above 75 percent on an acceleration, shorten your stride, keep the feet lower to the ground, avoid pushing off hard, and glide fast. This should keep the heart rate from getting out of bounds.

Pacing mile repeats

Your speed sessions of mile repeats will not only develop the endurance and speed needed for the marathon, but also, with the help of the heart monitor, give you the biofeedback necessary to improve form at the same time. Each mile repeat should be run only about 20 seconds faster per mile than your goal-marathon pace. By using a heart monitor, you can teach yourself to run more efficiently by improving your form so that you run more smoothly.

Let's say that, during the first two mile repeats, your heart rate goes up to between 75 and 80 percent of maximum. On the remaining mile repeats, maintain the same pace but try to keep the heart rate from going beyond 75 percent by running more efficiently.

By keeping your monitor on during the rest interval, you can tell when you have recovered enough to run another mile repeat. Wait until your heart rate has gone below 70 percent and then walk for at least another 100 meters or so after that. It's better to let the heart rate drop to below 65 percent of maximum, if possible. This extra rest will improve recovery.

Speedwork with a monitor

The heart rate monitor is one of the best biofeedback devices for improving form through efficiency. As always, the best environment for change is managed stress, and the monitor can tell you when to back off. If you are just starting speedwork, once a week is often enough. Veteran speed trainers may do a second, but shorter, speed workout (or a race) during and leading up to racing season. Again, be sure to monitor your total workload and recovery from races, speed sessions, and long runs.

Venue

The best place for this speed workout is a track where you can monitor speed at a variety of short and longer intervals.

Distance

Start with the distance of an average run during the week.

The warm-up

Do at least 1 mile of easy jogging and half a mile of accelerations.

The workout

Run repetitions of between 800 and 1,600 meters. Start each at (or slightly below) your current race pace for the distance you have trained for so far. Increase the intensity until you are working at 70 percent of maximum heart rate but it should still feel natural and comfortable. Very gradually, increase to 80 percent of maximum. Now you're ready for the workout. Your goal is to find form improvements that will allow you to run faster yet stay at 80 percent of your maximum heart rate (or below).

Techniques

Shorten your stride an inch or two and increase turnover of your feet and legs. Keep the push-off short and quick and directly under the body. Shift between different muscle groups as necessary so that one group doesn't get tired.

Monitoring

While you are monitoring your heart rate, time segments on the track of 200 to 400 meters at a time. When the distance of the repetition gets too long (often somewhere between 800 and 1,200 meters), your heart rate will increase. This is a sign for you to take a break. Jog or walk to recover and start again.

The warm-down

This should involve at least 1 mile of slow jogging and 5 minutes of walking.

29 BEST FOOT FORWARD

The best advice in choosing a running shoe is to get the best advice—at an authentic running store.

Most runners collect a closet full of bargain shoes until they find a real running store. The good advice of a trained staff can cut through the conflicting information, match you up with current helpful technology, and help you find a shoe that becomes an extension of your foot. Few aspects of life change as rapidly as running shoes. Some of the changes are fueled by new technology. Most, unfortunately, are generated by the sales hype of companies competing for sales to a growing army of new runners.

Advantages of a good running store

1. Even the better companies are using gimmicks in their design. Some of the gimmicks work, and some don't.

2. There's always a reason that a catalogue offers a dramatic discount on a given shoe.

3. Shoes of the same style may be made in different factories and thus be significantly different in the way they fit and in the many subtle ways they work when you run.

4. Only sales people who are real runners keep up with the gossip about running shoes. They get constant feedback each week from hundreds of customers who really use the shoes for exercise.

5. Only experienced running-shoe salespeople can look at you running in a shoe and tell whether it really fits—and works with your foot in the right way.

Although they are rare, authentic running stores are managed and staffed by adult runners who make it their life to test shoes, learn about the action of the foot, and collect continuous feedback on what shoes really work. That's why I opened my running store, Phidippides, in 1973. I still own the store but my other activities keep me away most of the time. So now I, too, consult my staff each time I need a new pair of shoes. They haven't been wrong yet! If you're in Atlanta, please drop by.

On your own

If you can't find a running specialty store, the following procedure will help you sift through the maze of running shoes. It's not as good as getting the advice of a runner/salesperson, but if you follow the procedures described below and use your best instincts, you're more likely to choose a shoe that will work for you. You'll also save time by not listening to the pitch of commission-driven salespeople or high school kids at stores that sell all types of sport shoes.

1. Take along your worn shoes, the socks you use, foot devices, etc.—everything you would use on a run. If you forgot to bring the socks that you use, buy a pair in the store that closely matches the thickness of your favorite ones. A good shoe expert can read the wear pattern on your shoes, which is the best indicator of how your foot functions. If you don't have the resources of an expert available, look at the diagram below.

2. Remember, you're in charge. Sure, you want the best advice available, but you are the only one who can feel the shoe on your foot. Narrow down the selection and then run in each shoe. Eventually, you'll decide which works best for you as you run. Don't let anyone tell you that a specific shoe is the shoe for *you* if another shoe seems to feel better or more natural as you run. Get the best advice but then make up your own mind.

3. Be prepared to spend at least 45 minutes if necessary You'll be more likely to try out the various shoes available. Don't rush in and grab the same shoe you bought last year. In the shoe business production changes are made about every four months, so what may look like the same shoe often isn't. Besides, there's very likely to be a better one for your needs. Try out all of the options and then decide for yourself.

4. Provide the salesperson with helpful details: the terrain of your routes, your running schedule, injuries (particularly chronic ones), goals in the next six months, etc.

5. Get feedback. Ask the salespeople to define the word *over-pronation*. If they pass that test, ask them to watch you run in each shoe. As you feel how each one works, get feedback from your salesperson.

6. Look at function first and then go for fit. Once you've found at least two to three pairs of shoes that seem to function well on your foot, adjust the lacing to fine-tune the fit of each shoe.

7. Choose the shoe that works best when you run. As you run in each one of your final candidates, determine which fits your foot naturally and functions as an extension of your foot. If you still can't decide, ask the salesperson which one lasts longer and whether the store has had any feedback from customers about how well the shoes work a month or two down the road.

The don'ts of shoe selection

- Don't get a shoe because it has worked well for someone else.

- Don't select the shoe that best matches your outfit.

- Don't take too seriously the advice of someone who can't give you a good definition of *over-pronation*.

- Don't buy from a shoe store that won't let you run in the shoe before you buy it.

- Don't pick the first shoe offered—especially if the salesperson says, "Trust me, I *know* that's the best shoe for you."
- Don't buy from a store in which most of the staff probably can't vote yet.
- Don't buy from a salesperson who tells you about his or her running, best times, etc., but doesn't ask you about your foot problems, past shoe successes, and special needs.
- Don't buy a shoe only because it's the most expensive.
- Don't get locked into specific models or brands. After trying on one or two shoes of a certain brand, some runners assume that all of the shoes of that brand, until eternity, are made the same way. All the major brands have various lasts and shapes, designed to fit most runners, and new batches are introduced about every six months. (If you have access to a shoe expert, be open to his or her suggestions; shoe experts will cheerfully sort through the hundreds of models currently available to find the best match for your foot.)

Definitions

Pronation is the normal rolling in of the foot to a flat or neutral position as you walk or run, to absorb shock. Most of us land on the outside of the heel and roll quickly to the forefoot. Your foot pronates, or rolls inward, to a flat and stable position before rolling forward toward the toe.

Over-pronation is rolling beyond the flat or neutral position of the foot, and that can (but doesn't always) produce injury. Primarily as a result of the structure of leg and foot bones and tendons, the foot

continues to roll to the inside as you push off. This tendency usually over-rotates the knee but can also produce damage to the hip, shin, ankle, and forefoot. When the force of your body weight presses down on a support structure that is out of alignment, as occurs with over-pronation, the weak link in your body will become injured. If there is any wear on the inside of the forefoot, you are an over-pronator.

Supination is rolling to the outside of the foot, which is usually okay because the bones on the outside of the foot are designed to support body weight. This motion causes a problem only when the foot continues to roll outside excessively, stressing the tendons of the ankle and sometimes the outside of the knee. This over-supination motion is evidenced by excessive shoe wear on the outside of the shoe and little wear elsewhere.

Floppy or rigid feet

Feet naturally seem to be floppy or rigid. If your foot had hinges, like a door, the floppy foot would be hinged so that it rolls easily from side to side. The rigid foot moves forward and back more easily.

Floppy feet often strike the ground first on the outside of the heel but, as the body moves forward, they roll to the inside. With this type of foot shoes usually show wear in spots, including some on the inside of the forefoot. Runners with rigid feet tend to push off forward strongly on the ball of the foot, and their shoes show wear on the outside of the forefoot as well as the middle.

Sometimes runners have one foot that's floppy and one that's rigid. Whatever type of foot you seem to have, there's no need to worry about it if you're not having aches, pains, or injuries. Your feet generally adapt so that you don't get injured as a result of your specific motion pattern. But the increased stress caused by increased mileage, speed training, or not enough days per week off from running can all tip the scales toward injury.

Runners with floppy feet should get a stable shoe, one that provides the foot with a good platform (this usually means minimal cushioning in the forefoot). There are shoes specifically designed for motion control and orthotic and other foot devices that reduce the chance of excessive rolling to the inside as the foot pushes off. Such devices can often help over-pronators who have chronic problems caused by alignment, but talk to a doctor before putting anything in your shoe.

Shape

The *last* of a shoe is the mold around which the shoe is built. If you look at the sole of a shoe that has a *curved last*, you will see not only a noticeable indention on the inside middle of the arch, but also that it actually curves so that the forefoot is given more support on the inside. When you look at a shoe with a *straight last*, however, the left shoe looks very similar to the right one. Most shoes today are made with elements of both the curved and the straight last. If a shoe puts pressure on the outside of your foot and there's extra room on the inside, you are trying on a shoe that is too curved for your foot. Ask to see a straighter one. If a shoe seems to put pressure on your big toe and joint, you need a shoe that is more curved.

Your foot should feel comfortable, naturally surrounded and protected—but not pushed up or pressured. The support of the shoe should be offered naturally so that you barely feel it. Never buy a shoe if it pinches or rubs parts of your feet when running. You know you've got a great fit when you run in the shoe and don't feel the shoe at all. Don't expect to get this perfect fit every time.

Lace that shoe securely

Many runners don't bother to pull the laces tight when they try on a shoe. A loose fit at the ankle is then mistaken for an ill-fitting heel. If there is excessive heel motion, pull the last few laces snug and tie the lace together so that there is no gap right at the knot. This may take several attempts because a new nylon lace is slick and resists being knotted tightly.

When to buy another shoe

As soon as you know that a certain shoe fits and feels good when you are running, get another pair before the company discontinues it. Each week, at the end of a run, put on the new pair and run around the block. Over the weeks, you'll break in the new pair. This procedure also provides a reality check of shoe support. After a month or so, you'll know when the original shoe needs to move on to greener pastures, perhaps as a lawn-mowing shoe. On that day, the new shoe gives support, while the old one flips, flops, and wobbles.

For more information on shoes, see *Galloway's Book on Running*.

MOVING THROUGH SPACE

"It's like a snowball rolling down the hill," says Ryan Lamppa, a researcher with the USA Track & Field Road Running Information Center in Santa Barbara, California. He refers to the "staggering" increase in marathon runners in recent years—451,000 finishers in U.S. marathons alone in 2000. "Virtually every major marathon in this country is selling out weeks in advance. With this pent-up demand, people sign-up as soon as the race opens its registration."

Why the growth?

"The marathon, the sport's Mt. Everest, has a special connotation in people's minds. It's a challenge, a sense of accomplishment that is different than running a 10K or half-marathon. Call it the marathon mystique."

Over the years, the marathon movement has created a lot of goodwill, which brings people back and draws new runners, and races today encourage people of all levels. Marathons are more inclusive than they used to be. For example, races keep the clocks going, so that whether you run 2:15 or 7:15, your time will still be recorded. (It wasn't that way in the past.) Also, there are kids' races along with the marathons, so that parents entering the races bring along their children, and the whole family has a running experience.

"Without question, with his training program, Jeff Galloway opened the door to 'average' people who didn't see themselves as marathoners, and the program's success rate speaks for itself," says Lamppa. "While another catalyst was Oprah Winfrey completing the Marine Corps Marathon in 1994 —which made headlines cross the country. Her exposure, busy schedule and body type caused people to think 'If Oprah can do it, so can I.' In short, Oprah inspired people—particularly women—to try running, and her impact still resonates today.

"It's also a social phenomenon. People see their friends running marathons and they ask 'How did you do it?'" It's now so easy to get information on training programs, he points out. "A search on the internet and a few clicks on a website or a phone call can get any information you need to run a marathon."

And as to the future, Lamppa points to the fact that there are 49 million kids under age 19 in the U.S. right now. This demographic group, called the "Echo Babies," is as big as the baby boomers and he feels that when they get to the median running age, the numbers of runners will increase even further.

"People are meant to run, to move through space." And the marathon is the perfect vehicle for our natural inclination.

APPENDIX

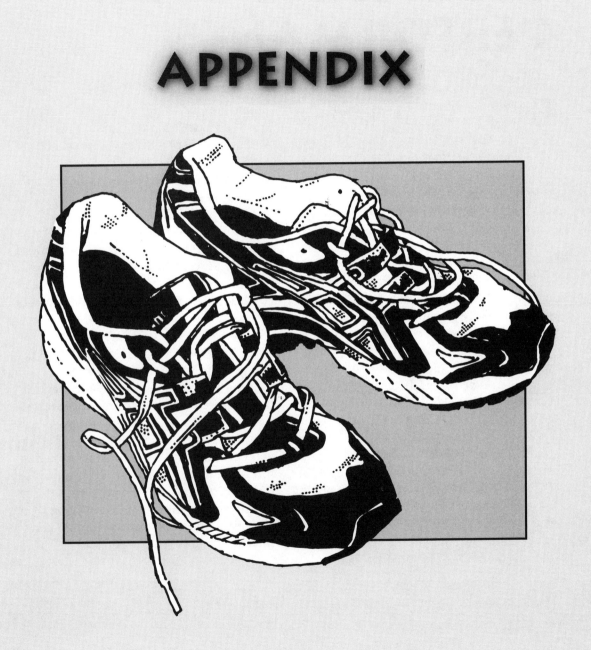

PREDICTING YOUR PERFORMANCE

By running several 5K races during your marathon training, you can predict how fast you're capable of going in the marathon itself. The following chart was designed by Gerry Purdy and reprinted, in part, from information supplied for *Galloway's Book on Running*. More extensive charts are offered in Gerry's Computerized Running Training Programs, published by Track & Field News.

If you're running your first marathon, use this chart only to see what you could run if you were running to capacity. Then set your goal about two minutes per mile slower than that time. If your first marathon is slow and enjoyable (the two conditions are related), you'll continue to enjoy exercise and benefit from it. You'll have the opportunity to run faster in the next marathon, or the one after that.

Run several 5Ks on weekends when you are not doing a long run. Make sure that they are run on certified courses, which have been accurately measured. See what your 5K predicts in the marathon. The more 5Ks you run, the better your prediction potential. The predictions on the charts are valid only if you have run the 26- to 28-mile training run (following the Two-Minute Rule) three weeks before the marathon itself. Those with goals of 3:40 and faster need to have also done the mile repeats as prescribed on the schedules beginning on p. 50.

If the marathon course is hilly or the temperature above 50 degrees F with more than 50 percent humidity, your time will not be as fast as it would be under ideal conditions. As the heat and humidity rise, you must adjust your pace to be more conservative from the first mile of the marathon. Be aware of heat disease symptoms and get help at the first sign of them.

This table is based upon ideal conditions, those that never occur together, so you must adjust it. Also, don't use your best 5K time to predict your marathon performance. Take an average of your three best times, and then add 10 to 20 minutes to the prediction. A conservative pace in the beginning will allow you to conserve your resources and enable you to run faster at the end if you're ready to do so.

PREDICTING RACE PERFORMANCE

5K Time (minutes)	Marathon Time (hours)	Half Marathon Time (hours)	5K Time (minutes)	Marathon Time (hours)	Half Marathon Time (hours)
13:20	2:10:00	1:01:24	16:57	2:47:05	1:18:37
13:25	2:10:46	1:01:45	17:04	2:48:21	1:19:12
13:29	2:11:32	1:02:06	17:12	2:49:38	1:19:48
13:34	2:12:19	1:02:28	17:19	2:50:56	1:20:24
13:38	2:13:06	1:02:50	17:27	2:52:15	1:21:01
13:43	2:13:54	1:03:13	17:35	2:53:36	1:21:38
13:48	2:14:43	1:03:35	17:43	2:54:58	1:22:16
13:53	2:15:32	1:03:58	17:51	2:56:21	1:22:54
13:58	2:16:22	1:04:22	17:59	2:57:45	1:23:33
14:03	2:17:12	1:04:46	18:07	2:59:11	1:24:13
14:08	2:18:04	1:05:09	18:15	3:00:39	1:24:53
14:13	2:18:55	1:05:33	18:24	3:02:07	1:25:34
14:18	2:19:48	1:05:57	18:32	3:03:37	1:26:16
14:23	2:20:41	1:06:22	18:41	3:05:09	1:26:58
14:28	2:21:34	1:06:47	18:50	3:06:42	1:27:41
14:34	2:22:29	1:07:13	18:59	3:08:17	1:28:24
14:39	2:23:24	1:07:38	19:08	3:09:53	1:29:09
14:44	2:24:20	1:08:04	19:18	3:11:32	1:29:54
14:50	2:25:16	1:08:30	19:27	3:13:11	1:30:40
14:56	2:26:13	1:08:57	19:37	3:14:53	1:31:27
15:01	2:27:11	1:09:24	19:47	3:16:36	1:32:14
15:07	2:28:10	1:09:51	19:57	3:18:21	1:33:02
15:13	2:29:10	1:10:18	20:07	3:20:08	1:33:52
15:19	2:30:10	1:10:47	20:17	3:21:57	1:34:42
15:25	2:31:11	1:11:15	20:27	3:23:48	1:35:33
15:31	2:32:13	1:11:44	20:38	3:25:41	1:36:25
15:37	2:33:16	1:12:13	20:49	3:27:36	1:37:18
15:43	2:34:20	1:12:42	21:00	3:29:34	1:38:11
15:49	2:35:25	1:13:13	21:11	3:31:33	1:39:07
15:55	2:36:30	1:13:43	21:23	3:33:35	1:40:02
16:02	2:37:37	1:14:14	21:34	3:35:39	1:40:59
16:08	2:38:44	1:14:45	21:46	3:37:46	1:41:57
16:15	2:39:53	1:15:17	21:58	3:39:55	1:42:56
16:22	2:41:02	1:15:49	22:10	3:42:06	1:43:57
16:29	2:42:13	1:16:22	22:23	3:44:21	1:44:57
16:36	2:43:24	1:16:54	22:36	3:46:38	1:46:00
16:43	2:44:37	1:17:28	22:49	3:48:58	1:47:05
16:50	2:45:50	1:18:03			

PREDICTING RACE PERFORMANCE (cont'd)

5K Time (minutes)	Marathon Time (hours)	Half Marathon Time (hours)	5K Time (minutes)	Marathon Time (hours)	Half Marathon Time (hours)
23:02	3:51:21	1:48:10	30:02	5:08:15	2:23:01
23:16	3:53:46	1:49:17	30:25	5:12:34	2:24:59
23:30	3:56:15	1:50:24	30:49	5:17:01	2:26:59
23:44	3:58:47	1:51:33	31:13	5:21:36	2:29:01
23:58	4:01:23	1:52:45	31:38	5:26:19	2:31:08
24:13	4:04:02	1:53:57	32:05	5:31:12	2:33:30
24:28	4:06:44	1:55:11	32:31	5:36:17	2:36:00
24:43	4:09:30	1:56:26	32:59	5:41:23	2:38:30
24:59	4:12:20	1:57:44	33:28	5:46:50	2:41:00
25:15	4:15:13	1:59:03	33:55	5:51:58	2:43:30
25:31	4:18:11	2:00:24	34:19	5:56:01	2:46:00
25:47	4:21:13	2:01:47	34:48	6:01:24	2:48:00
26:04	4:24:19	2:03:11	35:05	6:05:00	2:49:00
26:22	4:27:29	2:04:37	35:30	6:10:00	2:51:00
26:40	4:30:45	2:06:06	35:55	6:15:00	2:53:00
26:58	4:34:05	2:07:36	36:20	6:20:00	2:55:00
27:16	4:37:30	2:09:09	36:45	6:25:00	2:57:00
27:35	4:41:00	2:10:44	37:10	6:30:00	2:59:00
27:55	4:44:36	2:12:22	37:35	6:35:00	3:01:00
28:15	4:48:17	2:14:02	38:00	6:40:00	3:03:00
28:35	4:52:04	2:15:44	38:25	6:45:00	3:05:00
28:56	4:55:57	2:17:29	38:50	6:50:00	3:07:00
29:18	4:59:56	2:19:18	39:15	6:55:00	3:09:00
29:39	5:04:02	2:21:08	39:45	7:00:00	3:11:00

PACE CHART

Mile	2-mile	5-mile	10-mile	13-mile	Half Marathon	15-mile	20-mile	Marathon
5:00	10:00	25:00	50:00:00	1:05:00	1:05:30	1:15:00	1:40:00	2:11:00
5:20	10:40	26:40	53:20:00	1:09:20	1:09:52	1:20:00	1:46:40	2:19:44
5:40	11:20	28:20	56:40:00	1:13:40	1:14:14	1:25:00	1:53:20	2:28:28
6:00	12:00	30:00	1:00:00	1:18:00	1:18:36	1:30:00	2:00:00	2:37:12
6:20	12:40	31:40	1:03:20	1:22:20	1:22:58	1:35:00	2:06:40	2:45:56
6:40	13:20	33:20	1:06:40	1:26:40	1:27:20	1:40:00	2:13:20	2:54:40
7:00	14:00	35:00	1:10:00	1:31:00	1:31:42	1:45:00	2:20:00	3:03:24
7:20	14:40	36:40	1:13:20	1:35:20	1:36:04	1:50:00	2:26:40	3:12:08
7:40	15:20	38:20	1:16:40	1:39:40	1:40:26	1:55:00	2:33:20	3:20:52
8:00	16:00	40:00	1:20:00	1:44:00	1:44:48	2:00:00	2:40:00	3:29:36
8:20	16:40	41:40	1:23:20	1:48:20	1:49:10	2:05:00	2:46:40	3:38:20
8:40	17:20	43:20	1:26:40	1:52:40	1:53:32	2:10:00	2:53:20	3:47:04
9:00	18:00	45:00	1:30:00	1:57:00	1:57:54	2:15:00	3:00:00	3:55:48
9:20	18:40	46:40	1:33:20	2:01:20	2:02:16	2:20:00	3:06:40	4:04:32
9:40	19:20	48:20	1:36:40	2:05:40	2:06:38	2:25:00	3:13:20	4:13:16
10:00	20:00	50:00	1:40:00	2:10:00	2:11:00	2:30:00	3:20:00	4:22:00
10:20	20:40	51:40	1:43:20	2:14:20	2:15:22	2:35:00	3:26:40	4:30:44
10:40	21:20	53:20	1:46:40	2:18:40	2:19:44	2:40:00	3:33:20	4:39:28
11:00	22:00	55:00	1:50:00	2:23:00	2:24:06	2:45:00	3:40:00	4:48:12
11:20	22:40	56:40	1:53:20	2:27:20	2:28:28	2:50:00	3:46:40	4:56:56
11:40	23:20	58:20	1:56:40	2:31:40	2:32:50	2:55:00	3:53:20	5:05:40
12:00	24:00	1:00:00	2:00:00	2:36:00	2:37:12	3:00:00	4:00:00	5:14:24
12:20	24:40	1:01:40	2:03:20	2:40:20	2:41:34	3:05:00	4:06:40	5:23:08
12:40	25:20	1:03:20	2:06:40	2:44:40	2:45:56	3:10:00	4:13:20	5:31:52
13:00	26:00	1:05:00	2:10:00	2:49:00	2:50:18	3:15:00	4:20:00	5:40:36
13:20	26:40	1:06:40	2:13:20	2:53:20	2:54:40	3:20:00	4:26:40	5:49:20
13:40	27:20	1:08:20	2:16:40	2:57:40	2:59:02	3:25:00	4:33:20	5:58:04
14:00	28:00	1:10:00	2:20:00	3:02:00	3:03:24	3:30:00	4:40:00	6:06:48
14:20	28:40	1:11:40	2:23:20	3:06:20	3:07:46	3:35:00	4:46:40	6:15:32
14:40	29:20	1:13:20	2:26:40	3:10:40	3:12:08	3:40:00	4:53:20	6:24:16
15:00	30:00	1:15:00	2:30:00	3:15:00	3:16:30	3:45:00	5:00:00	6:33:00
15:20	30:40	1:16:40	2:33:20	3:19:20	3:20:52	3:50:00	5:06:40	6:41:44
15:40	31:20	1:18:20	2:36:40	3:23:40	3:25:14	3:55:00	5:13:20	6:50:28
16:00	32:00	1:20:00	2:40:00	3:28:00	3:29:36	4:00:00	5:20:00	6:59:12
16:20	32:40	1:21:40	2:43:20	3:32:20	3:33:58	4:05:00	5:26:40	7:07:56
16:40	33:20	1:23:20	2:46:40	3:36:40	3:38:20	4:10:00	5:33:20	7:16:40
17:00	34:00	1:25:00	2:50:00	3:41:00	3:42:42	4:15:00	5:40:00	7:25:24
17:20	34:40	1:26:40	2:53:20	3:45:20	3:47:04	4:20:00	5:46:40	7:34:08
17:40	35:20	1:28:20	2:56:40	3:49:40	3:51:26	4:25:00	5:53:20	7:42:52
18:00	36:00	1:30:00	3:00:00	3:54:00	3:55:48	4:30:00	6:00:00	7:51:36

MAJOR MARATHONS

January

Walt Disney World® Marathon and Half Marathon
P.O. Box 10000
Lake Buena Vista, FL 32830
407-938-3398
www.disneyworldsports.com
course open 7 hours

Houston
720 North Post Oak Road
Suite 100
Houston, Texas 77024
713-957-3453
713-957-3406 (fax)
www.chevronhoustonmarathon.com
course open 6 hours

PF Chang's Rock 'n' Roll Arizona
Elite Racing
9401 Waples St., Suite 150
San Diego, CA 92121
800-311-1255
www.runrocknroll.competitor.com
course open 7:15 hours

Miami
US Road Sports & Entertainment of Florida, LLC
P.O. Box 56-1081
Miami, FL 33256
305-278-8668
www.ingmiamimarathon.com
course open 7 hours

February

Rock 'n' Roll New Orleans
Competitor Group
9401 Waples Street, Suite 150
San Diego, CA 92121
858-450-6510
858-450-6905 (fax)
www.runrocknroll.competitor.com
course open 7 hours

The Austin Marathon
P.O. Box 684587
Austin, TX 78768-4587
512-476-7223
www.youraustinmarathon.com
course open 7 hours

26.2 with Donna: The National Marathon to Fight Breast Cancer
2107 Mango Place
Jacksonville, FL 32207
904-355-PINK (7465)
www.breastcancermarathon.com
course open 7 hours

ING Georgia Marathon & Half Marathon
528 Plasters Ave NE
Atlanta, GA 30324
404-892-8383
404-892-8384 (fax)
www.inggeorgiamarathon.com
course open 7 hours

Los Angeles
9200 Sunset Blvd.
Ste. 520
Los Angeles, CA 90069
310-271-7200
310-271-7202 (fax)
www.lamarathon.com
no time limit

March

Albany, GA
112 N. Front Street
Albany, Georgia 31701
229-317-4760
229-317-4765 (fax)
www.albanymarathon.com/
course open 7 hours

April

Boston
Boston Athletic Association
105th Boston Marathon Race Application
"The Starting Line"/One Ash Street
Hopkinton, MA 01748-1897
617-236-1652
www.bostonmarathon.org
course open 6:15 hours

Big Sur
P.O. Box 222620
Carmel, CA 93922
831-625-6226
831-625-2119 (fax)
www.bsim.org
course open 6 hours

Country Music
220 Great Circle Rd., Suite. 134
Nashville, TN 37228
615-742-1660
615-742-1659 (fax)
www.runrocknroll.competitor.com
course open 7:30 hours

London
P.O. Box 1234
London SE1 8RZ
44 171 620 4117
44 171 620 4208 (fax)
www.virginlondonmarathon.com

Paris
Amaury Sport Organisation
2 rue Rouget de Lisle TSA 61100
92137 Issy-les-Moulineaux Cedex
+ (33) (0)1 41 33 14 00
+ (33) (0)1 41 33 14 29 (fax)
www.parismarathon.com

May

Cincinnati Flying Pig Marathon
644 Linn Street, Suite 626,
Cincinnati, OH, 45203
513-721-7447
www.flyingpigmarathon.com
course open 7 hours

Pittsburgh
425 Sixth Avenue Suite 1100
Pittsburgh, PA 15219-1811
412-392-1021
www.pittsburghmarathon.com
course open 7 hours

June

Rock 'n' Roll Marathon San Diego
c/o Elite Racing
9401 Waples St., Suite 150
San Diego, CA 92121
800-311-1255
www.runrocknroll.competitor.com
course open 7 hours

Rock 'n' Roll Seattle
Elite Racing Inc.
c/o Rock 'n' Roll Seattle
9401 Waples Street, Suite 150
San Diego, CA 92121
800-311-1255
858-450-6905 (fax)
www.unrocknroll.competitor.com
course open 7 hours

Grandma's Marathon
P.O. Box 16234
Duluth, Minnesota 55816
218-727-0947
218-727-7932 (fax)
www.grandmasmarathon.com
course open 6 hours

July

San Francisco
RunSFM
P.O. Box 77148
San Francisco, CA 94107
888-958-6668
www.runsfm.com
course open 5:30 hours

August

Humpy's Marathon
Anchorage Running Club
Humpy's Marathon
P.O. Box 243362
Anchorage, AK 99524-3362
www.humpysmarathon.com/
course open 7 hours

September

Berlin
SCC-RUNNING
Glockenturmstr. 23
14055 Berlin
49 30 / 30 12 88 - 10
49 30 / 30 12 88 - 20 (fax)
www.real-berlin-marathon.com
course open 6:15 hours

October

Portland Marathon
P.O. Box 4040
Beaverton, Oregon 97076
503.226.1111
www.portlandmarathon.org
course open 7:30 hours

Bank of America Chicago Marathon
135 S. LaSalle St., Suite 2705
MC: IL4-135-27-05
Chicago, IL 60603
312-904-9800
312-904-9820 (fax)
www.chicagomarathon.com
course open 6:30 hours

Medtronic Twin Cities Marathon
4050 Olson Memorial Highway
Suite 26.2
Minneapolis, MN 55422
763-287-3888
763-287-3889 (fax)
www.twincitiesmarathon.org
course open 6 hours

Marine Corps Marathon
P.O. Box 188
Quantico, VA 22134
1-800-RUN USMC
703-784-2265 (fax)
www.marinemarathon.com

Des Moines Marathon
4801 Grand Avenue
Des Moines, Iowa 50312
515-288-2692
515.225.9051 (fax)
www.desmoinesmarathon.com
course open 7 hours

BassPro Springfield
1935 S. Campbell
Springfield, MO 65807
417-891-5214
www.basspro.com
course open 8 hours

St. George Marathon
86 South Main
St. George, UT 84770
435-627-4500
435-627-4509 (fax)
www.stgeorgemarathon.com

Hartford Marathon Foundation
140 Hebron Ave.
Glastonbury, CT 06033
860-652-8866
860-652-8145 (fax)
www.hartfordmarathon.com
course open 6 hours

November

Athens, Greece
www.athensmarathon.com

ING New York City Marathon
New York Road Runners
9 East 89th Street
New York, NY 10128
212-423-2249
www.nycmarathon.org
course open 8:20 hours

Rock 'n' Roll San Antonio
Competitor Group
c/o Rock 'n' Roll San Antonio
9401 Waples Street, Suite 150
San Diego, CA 92121
800-311-1255
858-450-6905 (fax)
www.runrocknroll.competitor.com
course open 7:30 hours

Space Coast – Melbourne, FL
Running Zone, Inc.
3680 N. Wickham Road, Unit C
Melbourne, FL 32935
321-751-8890
321-751-8890 (fax)
www.spacecoastmarathon.com
course open 7 hours

Philadelphia Marathon
Memorial Hall
4231 North Concourse Drive
Philadelphia, PA 19131
215-685-0054
215-685-0061 (fax)
www.philadelphiamarathon.com
course open 7 hours

December

Rock 'n' Roll Las Vegas
Competitor Group
9401 Waples St.
Suite 150
San Diego, CA 92121
858-450-6510
858-450-6905 (fax)
www.runrocknroll.competitor.com
course open 7 hours

Thunder Road – Charlotte, NC
Run for Your Life
2422 Park Rd.
Charlotte, N. C. 28203
704-358-0717
www.runcharlotte.com
course open 6 hours

California International Marathon
120 Ponderosa Ct.
Folsom, CA 95630
916-983-4622
916-983-4624 (fax)
www.runcim.org
course open 6 hours

Dallas White Rock Marathon
4950 Keller Springs Road, Suite 240
Addison, TX 75001
972-839-3976
214-376-4675 (fax)
www.runtherock.com
course open 6:30 hours

Honolulu Marathon
3435 Waialae Avenue, Room 200
Honolulu, Hawaii 96816
808-734-7200
808-732-7057 (fax)
www.honolulumarathon.org
course open 9 hours

Other great resources for race info, runner reviews, courses and profiles are *www.marathonguide.com* and *www.runnersworld.com*.

Note: Marathon data is updated every 3 months. For the latest info, see www.RunInjuryFree.com.

RUNNING RESOURCES AND CONTACTS

UNITED STATES

Alaska

Skinny Raven Sports
800 H Street
Anchorage, AK 99501
www.skinnyraven.com

Arizona

***Jeff Galloway Training Program*™**
Phoenix, Tucson
www.JeffGalloway.com

Arkansas

Fleet Feet – Fayetteville
1020 Harold Street
Fayetteville, AK 72703
www.fleetfeetfayetteville.com/

Gearhead Outfitters
230 South Main Street
Jonesboro, AK 72401
www.gearheadoutfitters.com/header.html

Gellco Outdoors
4600 South Zero
Ft. Smith, AK 72903
www.gellcooutdoors.com

The Sporty Runner
1016 Van Ronkle Street
Conway, AK 72032
www.thesportyrunner.com

California

***Jeff Galloway Training Program*™**
Inland Empire, Los Angeles, Orange County, San Jose
www.JeffGalloway.com

Athletic Performance
1115 Lincoln Avenue
San Jose, CA 95125
www.athleticperformancesanjose.com

Fleet Feet – Sacramento
2311 J Street
Sacramento, CA 95816
www.fleetfeetsacramento.com/

Sierra Running Company
9447 N. Fort Washington, #106
Fresno, CA 93720
www.sierrarunco.com

Colorado

***Jeff Galloway Training Program*™**
Boulder, Denver
www.JeffGalloway.com

Fleet Feet – Boulder
2624 Broadway
Boulder, CO 80304
www.fleetfeetboulder.com/

Runner's Roost
1685 South Colorado Blvd., Unit J
Denver, CO 80222
www.runnersroost.com

Connecticut

***Jeff Galloway Training Program*™**
Hartford
www.JeffGalloway.com

Florida

***Jeff Galloway Training Program*™**
Daytona, Ft. Lauderdale, Jacksonville, Lakeland, Navarre Beach, Orlando, Pensacola, Sarasota, St. Augustine, Stuart, Tallahassee, Tampa
www.JeffGalloway.com

Fleet Feet – Stuart
2440 NW Federal Highway
Stuart, FL 34994
www.fleetfeetstuart.com/

Run With It
1888 Andorra Street
Navarre, FL 32566
www.runwithitnavarre.com

Running Zone, Inc.
3708 N. Wickham Road
Melbourne, FL 32935
www.runningzone.com

Team Footworks
5724 Sunset Drive
South Miami, FL 33143
www.teamfootworks.org

The Running Center
14308 North Dale Mabry Hwy, #E
Tampa, FL 33618
www.runcenter.com

The Track Shack
1104 N. Mills Avenue
Orlando, FL 32803
www.trackshack.com

Georgia
Jeff Galloway Training Program™
Atlanta, Albany, Gwinnett, Macon, North Gwinnett, Savannah
www.JeffGalloway.com

Phidippides
1544 Piedmont Road
Atlanta, GA 30324
www.phidippides.com

Phidippides
220 Sandy Springs Circle
Atlanta, GA 30328
www.phidippides.com

Hawaii
Jeff Galloway Training Program™
Oahu
www.JeffGalloway.com

Running Room–Hawaii
819 Kapahula Avenue
Honolulu, HI 96816
www.runningroomhawaii.com

Idaho
Jeff Galloway Training Program™
Jerome
www.JeffGalloway.com

Bandana Running & Walking
504 W Main Street
Boise, ID 83702
www.bandannarunning.com

Illinois
Jeff Galloway Training Program™
Chicago, Hinsdale
www.JeffGalloway.com

The Runner's Edge
335 Ridge Road
Wilmette, IL 60091
www.runswim.com

Urban Tri Gear
210 Burr Ridge Parkway
Burr Ridge, IL 60527
www.urbantrigear.com

Indiana
Jeff Galloway Training Program™
Indianapolis West, Valparaiso
www.JeffGalloway.com

Louisiana
Jeff Galloway Training Program™
Natchitoches
www.JeffGalloway.com

Maryland
Jeff Galloway Training Program™
Annapolis, Baltimore
www.JeffGalloway.com

Fleet Feet Sports–Baltimore
1809 Reisterstown Road
Baltimore, MD 21208
www.fleetfeetbaltimore.com/

Massachusetts
Bill Rodgers Running Center
353-T North Market Place
Boston, MA 02109
www.billrodgers.com

Maine
Maine Running Company
563 Forest Avenue
Portland, ME 04101
www.mainerunning.com/

Michigan
Jeff Galloway Training Program™
Lupton–Northern Michigan
www.JeffGalloway.com

The Complete Runner
915 S. Dort Highway, #F
Flint, MI 48503
www.thecompleterunner.com/

Mississippi
Jeff Galloway Training Program™
Greenville
www.JeffGalloway.com

Missouri
Jeff Galloway Training Program™
Springfield
www.JeffGalloway.com

Garry Gribble Running Sports
18810 E 39th Street
Independence, MO 64057
www.garrygribbles.com

Garry Gribble Running Sports
8600 Ward Parkway
Kansas City, MO 64114
www.garrygribbles.com

Montana
Time Out Sports
1603 Grand Avenue
Billings, MT 59102
www.timeoutsports.biz

Nebraska
Confluence
505 Cornhusker Road, #107
Bellevue, NE 68005
www.confluencebookstore.com

Nevada
Scheels
1200 Scheels Drive
Sparks, NV 89434
www.scheelssports.com

New Jersey
*Jeff Galloway Training
  Program*™
Mahwah
www.JeffGalloway.com

Shore Runner
40 Centennial Drive
Long Branch, NJ 07740
www.shorerunner.com

New Mexico
*Jeff Galloway Training
  Program*™
Albuquerque,
  Artesia–Southeastern NM
www.JeffGalloway.com

ABQ Running Shop
12611 Montgomery Blvd., NE,
A6-B
Albuquerque, NM 87111
www.abqrunningshop.com

New York
*Jeff Galloway Training
  Program*™
New York
www.JeffGalloway.com

North Carolina
*Jeff Galloway Training
  Program*™
Charlotte, Charlotte–Lake
  Norman, Raleigh
www.JeffGalloway.com

North Dakota
*Jeff Galloway Training
  Program*™
Fargo
www.JeffGalloway.com

Scheels
1551 45th Street SW
Fargo, ND 58103
www.scheelssports.com

Ohio
*Jeff Galloway Training
  Program*™
Cincinnati
www.JeffGalloway.com

Oregon
*Jeff Galloway Training
  Program*™
Eugene
www.JeffGalloway.com

Pennsylvania
*Jeff Galloway Training
  Program*™
Philadelphia
www.JeffGalloway.com

Fleet Feet–North Wales
1210 Bethlehem Pike
North Wales, PA 19454
www.fleetfeetnorthwales.com

Philadelphia Runner
1601 Sansom Street
Philadelphia, PA 19103
www.philadelphiarunner.com

The Running Place
3548 Westchester Pike
Newtown Square, PA 19073
www.therunningplace.com

South Carolina
*Jeff Galloway Training
  Program*™
Hartsville
www.JeffGalloway.com

Tennessee
*Jeff Galloway Training
  Program*™
Nashville, Tennessee Valley
www.JeffGalloway.com

Texas
*Jeff Galloway Training
  Program*™
Austin, Bryan/College Station,
  Coppell, Dallas, El Paso,
  Fort Worth, Houston,
  New Branufels, Temple, Waco
www.JeffGalloway.com

Finish Line Sports
13895 SW Freeway
Sugarland, TX 77478
slfinishlinesports.com

Utah
*Jeff Galloway Training
  Program*™
Salt Lake City
www.JeffGalloway.com

Salt Lake Running Company
3142 S Highland Drive–A-5
Salt Lake City, UT 84106
*www.saltlakerunningco.com/
saltlake*

Vermont
*Jeff Galloway Training
  Program*™
Burlington
www.JeffGalloway.com

Virginia
*Jeff Galloway Training
  Program*™
Hampton Roads
www.JeffGalloway.com

Washington, D.C.
*Jeff Galloway Training
  Program*™
Metro DC
www.JeffGalloway.com

Wisconsin
*Jeff Galloway Training
  Program*™
Milwaukee
www.JeffGalloway.com

PUERTO RICO

Jeff Galloway Training Program™

Guaynabo
www.JeffGalloway.com

CANADA

Jeff Galloway Training Program™

Surrey, BC
www.JeffGalloway.com

Bialkowski Try Sport

77 Bowes Street
Parry Sound, ON P2A 2L6
www.ontariotrysport.com

Running Room Ltd.

9750 47th Avenue
Edmonton, AL T6E 5P3
www.runningroom.com

ITALY

Jeff Galloway Training Program™

Milan
www.JeffGalloway.com

Other groups include the National AIDS Marathon Training Program, www.aidsmarathon.org, and the LA Leggers, www.laleggers.org.

Look for Jeff's articles at www.runnersworld.com.

Tawni Gomes is an on-line support group — www.connectingconnectors.com, 650-991-4200 — inspired by Oprah Winfrey and Bob Greene, author of Making the Connection.

Note: Running resources and contacts are updated every 3 months. For the latest info, see www.RunInjuryFree.com.

STATISTICS ON MARATHONS

In 2009, the U.S.A. Track and Field Road Running Information Center published race data from major U.S. races, showing the continuing growth of marathon runners, and sex and age of participants. Here are the statistics:

Number of Marathon Finishers in U.S.

Year	Estimated # of finishers
1976	25,000
1980	143,000
1990	224,000
1995	293,000
2000	353,000
2005	395,000
2008	425,000 (record total)

World's Largest Marathons (finishers)

Race	Finishers
1. New York	38,096
2. Berlin	35,746
3. London	34,603
4. Chicago	31,343
5. Paris	28,846
6. Tokyo	26,672
7. Boston	21,945
8. Honolulu	20,061
9. Naha (Japan)	18,654
10. Marine Corps, D.C.	18,228

Largest U.S. Marathons (finishers)

Race	Finishers
1. New York, NY	38,096
2. Chicago, IL	31,343
3. Boston, MA	21,945
4. Honolulu, HI	20,061
5. Marine Corps, D.C.	18,228
6. Los Angeles, CA	17,247
7. Rock 'n' Roll, CA	16,873
8. Walt Disney World, FL	12,964
9. Twin Cities, MN	7,979
10. Portland, OR	7,879

Demographic Breakdown

	1980	1995	2000	2006	2008
Males	89.5%	74%	62%	60%	59%
Females	10.5%	26%	38%	40%	41%
Juniors	5%	2%	2%	2%	2%
Masters	26%	41%	44%	46%	45%

Median Age

	1980	1995	2000	2006	2008
Males	34	38	38	40	39
Females	31.3	35	35	35	35

Median Times for U.S. Marathon Finishers

	1980	1995	2002	2006	2008
Males	3:32:17	3:54:00	4:20:01	4:15:34	4:16:00
Females	4:03:39	4:15:00	4:56:46	4:46:40	4:43:32

ABOUT THE AUTHOR

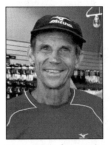 In the 1970s, Jeff Galloway was one of a group of young American runners who would change distance running forever. Jeff and his running buddies —Frank Shorter, Bill Rodgers, Steve Prefontaine, Don Kardong, Amby Burfoot, Kenny Moore, and others—captured the attention of a new generation of fitness-minded Americans, and the running boom was born. What had been a sport for the few became an activity for the millions.

Jeff was born in Raleigh, North Carolina, started running in the 8th grade, as a fat kid. Five years later he was was state champion in the 2-mile. He attended Wesleyan University and was All-American in cross-country and track. In preparing for the 1972 Olympics, Jeff, along with Frank Shorter and Jack Bacheler, spent two months training in the mountains at Vail, Colorado, and all three made the Olympic team that year. Jeff, according to runner/writer Joe Henderson "... should have been an Olympic marathoner, but instead made the team in the 10K and then helped friend Jack Bacheler make it in the longer distance."

In 1973 Jeff set an American record in the 10-mile. He won the first Atlanta Marathon at age 18, and was the first winner of Atlanta's Peachtree Road Race in 1970. In the mid-'70s he began to follow a training program that emphasized more rest and less weekly mileage, coupled with a long run every other week. At age 35 he ran the Houston-Tenneco Marathon in a personal lifetime record of 2:16.

Jeff Galloway's Competitive Career

High school:	1-mile: 4:28;	
	2-mile: 9:48	
College:	1-mile: 4:12;	
	2-mile: 9:06;	
	3-mile: 14:10	
Other times:	6-mile: 27:21	
	10K: 28:29	
	10-mile: 47:49	
	(U.S. record, 1973)	

Jeff met his wife Barbara at the Florida State track. Barbara was on the FSU women's track team. They were married in 1976. Barbara runs practically every day and has competed in over 70 marathons. Her best 10K time is 41:50 and marathon time, 3:18.

Jeff is now on the road over half the time. Because of his busy schedule, he often runs 2–5 miles, two or three times per day. He generally totals about 40 miles a week. He has currently run 150 marathons, at the rate of 6–7 per year. Every ten years he returned to the site of his first victory, Atlanta, and beat his time of 2:56 as an 18-year-old. In 1993, at age 48, he ran just under 2:51.

Jeff and Barbara live in Atlanta, Georgia and their beach retreat: Blue Mountain Beach, Florida. Their two adult sons, Brennan and Westin, like their parents, are (naturally!) runners.

Jeff Galloway Online

Website: www.JeffGalloway.com

Blog: www.JeffGallowayBlog.com

Twitter: www.twitter.com/jeffgalloway

Facebook: www.facebook.com/JeffGalloway

Fan Page: www.facebook.com/JeffGallowayfan

LinkedIn: www.linkedin.com/in/jeffgalloway

INDEX

GALLOWAY'S TRAINING GROUPS IN 72 MAJOR CITIES
Getting to the finish line injury-free

The group guides you, encourages you, and supports you during your 6-month training program. There are currently groups in the following cities:

Albany, GA	Eugene, OR	Mahwah, NJ	Puerto Rico
Albuquerque, NM	Fargo, ND	Metro DC	Raleigh, NC
Annapolis, MD	Fort Lauderdale,	Program	Salt Lake City, UT
Atlanta, GA	FL	Milan, Italy	San Jose, CA
Austin, TX	Fort Worth, TX	Milwaukee, WI	Sarasota, FL
Baltimore, MD	Greenville, MS	N. Gwinnett, GA	Savannah, GA
Boston, MA	Gwinnett Co., GA	Nashville, TN	Southeastern New
Boulder, CO	Hampton Roads,	Natchitoches, LA	Mexico
Bryan/College	VA	Navarre Beach, FL	Springfield, MO
Station, TX	Hartford, CT	New Braunfels,	St.Augustine, FL
Burlington, VT	Hartsville, SC	TX	Stuart, FL
Charlotte - Lake	Hinsdale, IL	New York, NY	Surrey, BC
Norman, NC	Houston, TX	Northern	Canada
Charlotte, NC	Indianapolis West,	Michigan	Tallahassee, FL
Chicago, IL	IN	Oahu, HI	Tampa, FL
Cincinnati, OH	Inland Empire, CA	Orange County,	Temple, TX
Coppell, TX	Jacksonville, FL	CA	Tennessee Valley,
Dallas, TX	Jerome, ID	Orlando, FL	TN
Daytona, FL	Lakeland, FL	Pensacola, FL	Tucson, AZ
Denver , CO	Los Angeles, CA	Philadelphia, PA	Valparaiso, IN
El Paso, TX	Macon, GA	Phoenix, AZ	Waco, TX

Not in a city near you? No problem. Join our Individual Training Program. Enjoy the guidance of a trained Virtual Group Leader. For more information:

www.RunInjuryFree.com
1-800-200-2771, ext 12

THE RUNNING NEWSLETTER

Stay in touch with the latest running ideas and concepts with Jeff's free monthly email newsletter. Training, fat-burning, marathon gatherings, and runner feedback.

To sign up for this FREE newsletter, call 1-800-200-2771 or go to www.JeffGalloway.com

JEFF'S COLUMN IN RUNNER'S WORLD

Read Jeff Galloway's monthly column in *Runner's World* magazine (www.RunnersWorld.com).

JEFF'S E-COACHING

This Individual "e-Coaching" Program gives you a training program designed by Jeff and direct, priority access to him when you have questions or clarifications. Whether you just want to run without pain, or qualify for the Boston Marathon, we will provide you with 6 months of coaching support, a training program suited for your goal, and many other items. This program is for all levels of runners, including beginners. Jeff's overall training philosophy is to provide you with a program toward your goals while "having a life," family, career. At every level, Jeff recommends lower mileage, fewer days per week, walk breaks.

Over the years, over 98% of his participants have successfully finished marathons and had similar success rates at other distances. Not only can you set up and record your progress for a year at a time, you'll be able to analyze the data in tables: logs for shoes, injuries, and speed sessions. Graphs for monitoring your pulse will help you avoid overtraining.

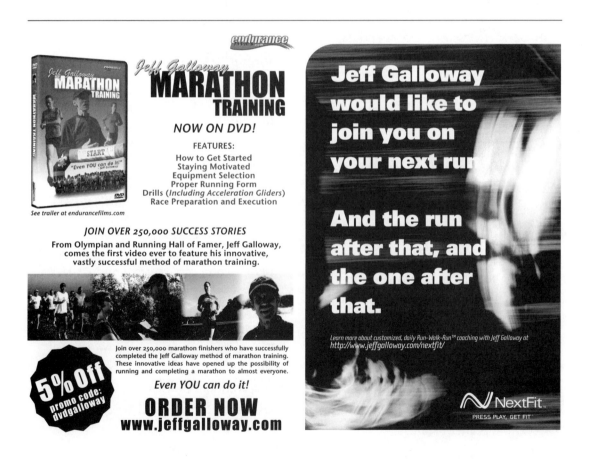

RE-ENERGIZE YOUR RUNNING
Lake Tahoe July Fitness Vacation

Join Jeff and his guests for a week or weekend in beautiful Squaw Valley, on the north shore of Lake Tahoe.

- Invited guests include:

   Joe Henderson – running's most prolific writer who knows just about everything that's going on in our sport

   Sister Marion Irvine – the humorous and inspiring nun who qualified for the Olympic Trials at age 50

   Dr. Gary Moran – physiologist and expert in biomechanics, strength, etc.

   Dr. David Hannaford – sports podiatrist specializing in running injuries

- Everyone stays at the comfortable and beautiful Squaw Valley Lodge, with hot tubs, swimming, tennis, health club, etc.

- Retreat starts at 5:00 p.m. on Friday with an easy run to get acquainted.

- Each morning starts with a run or walk, whichever you choose (optional, of course), breakfast and then clinics by Jeff and his guests. Ask all the questions you wish.

- After lunch, you may shop, sight-see, sun by the pool or join the group for a scenic hike, T-shirt swap, etc.

- The group (@40) gathers again in the evenings for dinner onsite or at one of the nearby restaurants and after-dinner relaxing.

- All meals are included except for Saturday, Sunday & Wednesday dinners.

- Checkout is after breakfast on the last day.

> For more info, contact
> carol.miller@JeffGalloway.com.

Florida Beach Retreat
Blue Mountain Beach, FL (near Destin)— for all levels

Jeff Galloway has helped over 250,000 runners and walkers reach their goals and can answer just about any training question. His motivational energy gets each participant involved in each session to provide the individual information needed.

- Individualized running form evaluation
- Nutrition & Fat-burning • Setting up a year-round program • Mental toughness & motivation • Running faster • Help with individualized goals • Priority email access afterward • Wonderful forest trails • Individualized help with running improvement

Running Schools
Hear Jeff speak about:

- **Extending Endurance**—without much fatigue, aches or pains

- **Getting Faster**—often when running fewer days per week or fewer miles per week

- **Staying Motivated**—training yourself to stay on track, get out the door, better mental toughness

- **Running Injury-Free**—stopping injuries before you limp, reducing injury risk to almost zero

- Nutritional information for your specific needs/problems

- Fatburning without being hungry all the time

- Inspirational Stories

- Extended direct email access to Jeff afterward

For five-hour sessions:

- Individualized running form evaluation
- Instruction in running form drills that make running easier

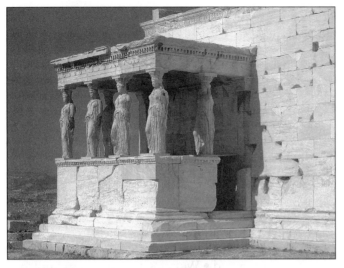

MORE WORLD-CLASS FITNESS BOOKS
FROM SHELTER PUBLICATIONS

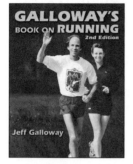

Galloway's Book on Running
2nd Edition
by Jeff Galloway

A complete revision of Jeff's classic book on running.

- 430,000 copies of original edition sold
- Training programs for 5K, 10K, and half marathons
- The second running boom
- New info on diet, "slow" running, clothing, and shoes

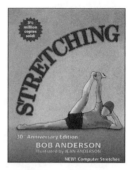

Stretching
30th Anniversary Revised Edition
by Bob Anderson

One of the world's most popular fitness books, now revised.

- 3½ million copies sold, in 23 languages
- Stretching routines for all sports (including running and everyday activities)
- 10 new stretching routines for office workers and computer operators

"A must-read for anyone who wants to stay supple for life."

–The Washington Post

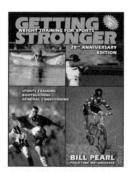

Getting Stronger
20th Anniversary Edition
by Bill Pearl

A revised edition of the best-seller on weight training. Of special interest to runners are off-season and in-season weight training programs for distance running and new rehab exercises for knees.

- 550,000 copies sold
- 80 one-page training programs
- General conditioning, sports training, and bodybuilding

"A must for anyone serious about fitness."

–Newsday

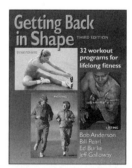

Getting Back in Shape:
32 Workout Programs for Lifelong Fitness
by Bob Anderson, Bill Pearl,
Ed Burke, and Jeff Galloway

A unique workout book for anyone who wants to get back in shape.

- Stretching, weightlifting, and cardiovascular training
- 3-point programs

". . . simple programs designed for the busy schedule."

–Kiplinger's Personal Finance magazine

CREDITS

Editors
Lloyd Kahn, Robert Lewandowski, Frances Bowles

Production Manager
Rick Gordon

Book Design
Rick Gordon, Lloyd Kahn, Robert Lewandowski, David Wills

Line Drawing Illustrations
David Wills

Photos
Joseph Sohm: Front and back covers, pp. 59, 77, 93, and 105
Jennifer Bailey: Title page
Rick Gordon: Photoshop special effects

Proofreading
Robert Grenier

Printing
Courier Companies, Inc., Stoughton, MA, USA

Production Hardware
Macintosh G5 computer, Agfa Arcus II scanner

Production Software
Adobe InDesign, Adobe Photoshop, Microsoft Word

Typefaces
Guardi, ITC Kabel, and Lithos

Paper
60 lb. Courier Offset

Special thanks to the following people, who helped with this book in one way or another:

John Cantwell, M.D., Leah Denney, Michele Langevin, Carol Miller, Victoria Seahorn, Don Shutters, Diana Twiggs, M.D.

FEEDBACK ON THE PROGRAMS IN THIS BOOK . . .

"I want to thank you for the most incredible, *unbelieveable* experience of my life. Never in a million years did I think I could accomplish such a feat. I have never done anything athletic in my entire life. I can't express how I felt going through the finish line at the NYC Marathon. I had so many emotions going through me, I almost lost my breath!"

–Jackie Baca,
New York City

"One of my goals in life was to run a marathon. With the Galloway Program, not only did I fulfill my dream, but I never thought I would be able to run four marathons in two years, injury-free. It not only changed the way I live but also changed my outlook on life: I take it one mile at a time."

–Jane Mun,
New York City

"Reading your article made it OK for me to walk during training runs, and during the marathon. I do not know if I would have been able to complete the marathon otherwise . . . Keep up your excellent work, and *never ever* stop talking about the run/walk plan. It makes the marathon accessible to people who would otherwise never dream of doing a marathon. It really works! Thank you so much!!!"

–Tim Esser

"I took the walk breaks, did the rubber-band trick, kept the brain positive and guess what? I qualified for Boston with a little time to spare. I think that of all the marathons I have ever done . . . this one meant the most of all to me. It does work. Thanks again."

–Patti Wathke,
Eau Claire, WI

"I am a 42-year-old homemaker in Roswell, GA, with a dream of some day running a marathon . . . I have been following your run/walk training schedule and I love it. I just ran/walked 9 miles on a beautiful Sunday morning and feel wonderful . . . I just *know* I can run/walk this half marathon now. You have been an enormous help in helping me work towards realizing my dream."

–Terry Phillips,
Roswell, GA

"Everyone is pulling for you to get to the finish line."

–Cesare Lucido